eanse ██████████████

Green Smoothie

Blueprint

A Comprehensive Guide in Detoxification and Cleansing Guide of Green Smoothies towards Optimum Health

Kate Philips
Copyright © Kate Philips

Plan for the day ahead. Think about what smoothies you are going to want to have the next day and prepare the ingredients the night before. You want to ensure that you do have all the necessary ingredients before you start to prepare your smoothies. The last thing you want to find out when you are getting ready in the morning is that you ran out of your favorite greens! 64

Introduction

When you think of a smoothie, you might picture a brightly colored beverage topped with whipped cream and served with a thick straw. While some restaurants may label these sugar-loaded beverages 'smoothies', they pale in comparison to real green smoothies.
A real, nutritious green smoothie is made using whole fruits and vegetables and not tainted by artificial sweeteners or unhealthy additives. Green smoothies are a great way to get your daily requirement of fruits and vegetables all in a tasty beverage.
If you are curious about what green smoothies are and how they can benefit you, keep reading! In this book, you will find valuable information regarding the benefits of green smoothies.
You need to clear out your body of toxins every so often because that's how you're going to increase the amount of health benefits that you have in your entire body. Those toxins that come about through your normal wear and tear of life are going to hurt your health. They're also going to increase your weight.

If you want to decrease your weight, green smoothie's can help you do that as well. Just take some time to focus on yourself. It will require you to reduce your intake of regular, traditional foods and focus on nutritious whole foods. Doing this will take planning. It requires you to concentrate. Simply follow the information we included in this book. Make sure that you include the right amount and type of smoothies in your daily diet. This process will allow you to cleanse your body and start yourself on a healthy path towards weight loss and health improvements. You'll just have to spend some time and some energy to achieve results.

Chapter 1

What is Green Smoothie Diet?

Proper Foods and Daily Exercise!

It's no secret to most that exercise and nutritious diet choices are the two main factors of health that we humans can control. It's our choice to be physically active or not on a daily basis, and it's also up to each of us to choose the right foods and beverages to deliver the nutrients we need to thrive. If we choose not to engage in physical activity or if we choose to ingest unhealthy food sources, then we are left to live less healthy lives than we could. Pretty simple really, right?

Hint: Green Smoothies make healthy food intake delicious, ultra-simple, and rewarding!

In most cases, people assume that getting and staying in control of their bodies is an incredibly complex matter. Some feel it is better left in the hands of physicians, nutritionist, and other types of medical experts, but that's not true! In fact, developing and maintaining increased health and fitness is a relatively straightforward matter.

Here are the two main points you need to accept:

1. You have to move your body by exercising on a daily basis.

2. You have to take in the nutrients that your body requires to function efficiently.

If you can accept the truth of these two guidelines, then you are already well on your way to achieving the health goals that have long eluded you.

It really is that easy!

For many people exercise is a dreaded act. Even though physical activity can be extremely enjoyable, there are those who just can't stand the thought of it! They may claim that they want to become more physically active, but they continually put off initiating an exercise plan. Likewise, many people erroneously believe that ensuring proper nutrition is an endeavor that will be unpleasant, distasteful, and difficult.

In my family, exercise is an accepted and expected element of our daily routines. It adds meaning, health, and enjoyment to all of our lives and we would live less fulfilled lives without it. It's the same now with Green Smoothies: everyone in the family loves their daily, tasty, and ultra-healthy Green Smoothies! Just drinking one each day becomes an enjoyable habit that you can be proud to add to your routine. You'll live a healthier, energy-filled, and natural lifestyle that will benefit everyone around you. Trust me! Best of all, it will benefit you the most!

A Brief History of Human Food Intake

Millions of years ago before industrialization, globalization, computerization, and urbanization, human beings were in much closer contact with the earth. There were no fast food joints to frequent, no organized governmental bodies dictating our food choices, and no political and economic motivations forcing people to live and eat in certain ways. In fact, there was just the need to survive. Food choices were quite limited according to an individual's location, climate conditions, and their abilities to successfully hunt and gather.

Obesity was seldom an issue for our prehistoric ancestors. Starvation was by far a larger concern. In general, the human diet consisted of natural plant products that people gathered. Occasionally, when a hunt went well, the animal products that were consumed were low in fat and without chemical additives like steroids, antibiotics, pesticides, herbicides, and other harmful substances. Everything was eaten fresh because there were no preservatives. Preservation methods involving chemicals had not been invented.

Approximately ten thousand years ago, agricultural practices surfaced across the planet, providing ready sources of grains, milk, potatoes, and other dietary staples. Additionally, the diversity of available meats and vegetables greatly increased. However, with this increased availability came issues of contamination, infestation, and more. People had to develop ways of protecting, storing, and preserving their food sources. Cooking became mainstream, and food preservation became a major societal concern.

As time passed, the world became more aware of the importance of food. Scientific minds questioned the ways in which foods affected us. Somewhere along the way, people started to understand the important relationship between our health and the foods we ate.

Fast Food History Facts!

- 400BC is when Hippocrates (the "Father of Modern Medicine") proclaimed: Let food be your medicine and medicine be your food!
- In the 16th century, Leonardo da Vinci compared human metabolism to a burning candle (a very accurate analogy!).
- In 1747, Dr. James Lind discovered that lime juice could spare British sailors from scurvy. Although the discovery continued to be ignored by the medical field for four decades to follow, British sailors eventually became known as "Limeys."

- During 1770, Antoine Lavoisier uncovered the fact that body heat is a result of food oxidation during digestion and assimilation.
- Carbon, nitrogen, oxygen, and hydrogen were recognized as the four main constituents of the foods we ate in the early part of the 19th century.
- In 1847, Justus Liebig reported that sugars make up carbohydrates, fatty acids were comprised of fats, and amino acid chains create proteins.
- In the 1860s, Claude Bernard proved that fat could be manufactured from proteins and carbohydrates. Thisdiscovery meant that blood glucose energy is able to be stored as either glycogen or fat.
- In the early 1900s, Carl Von Voit and Max Rubner both earned independent credit for first measuring the expenditure of energy in living organisms.
- In 1911, Casimir Funk combined the words "vital" & "amine" to form the word "vitamin."
- A year after that, Elmer McCollum discovered the first fat-soluble Vitamin A. He also discovered the first water-soluble vitamin B. (Of course, by 1915, Vitamin B "grew into" the Vitamin B complex, comprised of several different water-soluble vitamins.) Additionally, he finally gave a name to that mysterious substance that is known worldwide now for preventing scurvy: Vitamin C. (This guy liked to keep his naming simple!)

- During the 1930s, William Cumming Rose instructed us on essential amino acids, the building blocks of all-important protein.
- 1941 was the first year that an RDA (Recommended Daily Allowance) chart was established for vitamins.
- After the Industrial Revolution, various methods for storing and preserving food sources were created. These include milling, pressing, drying, cooling, heating, irradiating, and more. While these methods can be useful for cutting down on food-borne pathogens, they also partially deplete the nutritional values contained in foods.
- During the 1960s, families became less in touch with nature and became centered mainly in urban conglomerations. Two-income families became prevalent. People spent less time cooking and preparing healthy meals at home because of their busy life schedules. Fast food joints sprang up like weeds in the jungle – and obesity/disease rates began to skyrocket!
- Since then, you probably already know the rest of the story. Preventable diseases are at all-time high rates. Many studies state that more than a third of Americans are classified as "Obese."

Americans are putting themselves in serious danger because of the foods they choose!

It makes me so sad every time we travel to the city, we see all the people walking down the crowded sidewalks. So many people are obviously suffering, physically and emotionally because they're carrying far too much weight. They develop unhealthy eating habits and continue to make poor food intake decisions – and after years and years passing by, they find themselves experiencing various health problems, not knowing quite what to do about it.

I see all those people on the sidewalks, the looks of fatigue on their faces as they simply attempt to walk. I think of some of my long-time friends and about how they are literally falling apart physically. That's one of the biggest reasons I find it so easy to stay motivated about the Green Smoothie lifestyle. Every day, I see how Green Smoothies positively affect all of the different people that I know!

Even if everything else seems to be going wrong, we can all still blast our systems with raw, organic nutrients every day in the form of Green Smoothies and still come away feeling good. By drinking Green Smoothies, our minds are sharper, and we have more energy. This is because our bodies have been fortified with huge amounts of free radical destroying antioxidants and plenty of other nutrients. We're generally healthier from head to toe and that is a good thing no matter how you look at it!

Current Stats on American Health

- Average weight of US woman: Over 165 pounds.
- Average weight of US man: Over 195 pounds.
- Obesity is strongly correlated with almost every health concern, including various cancers, cardiovascular issues, diabetes, stroke, high blood pressure (hypertension), arthritis, and so many more.
- In 2009, health care costs in the US were approximately $2.47 trillion dollars. By 2019, that price tag is expected to rise up to about $4.5 trillion.
- Health care insurance rates have risen 300% faster than wages over the past 10 years.
- In 2009 alone, the top five health insurance companies in the US reported more than $12.2 billion in profits.

- In 2008, there were more than two dozen big pharmaceutical companies that made over 1 billion dollars in profit (each) from sales within the US.
- Nearly 50% of all Americans are on some type of regularly prescribed prescription medication.
- The majority of Americans are classified as "completely inactive" by health professionals from all fields.

Leading Causes of Death the US in

It's so sad when someone we know and love dies, but people do pass on and in so many cases, far too soon. It really makes me upset that so many people who die do so prematurely for no reason at all, except they just didn't remain committed to their own levels of health while they lived. Many smoke tobacco products, drink heavily, never exercise, eat high fat, high-sodium foods, and generally live like they want to die. What really gets to me is that many people seem oblivious to the fact that the majority of deaths by disease are completely preventable. Yes, preventable.

Even after someone is diagnosed with a specific disease or health condition, like colon cancer for example, they can still reverse the symptoms of the disease. In many cases, they can dissolve the malignancies completely by making positive lifestyle modifications that increase their overall health. According to the most recently published statistics from the Center for Disease Control (CDC), the leading causes of death in the US by percentages are:

- Heart disease: 24.5%
- Cancer: 23.3%
- Chronic lower respiratory diseases: 5.6%
- Stroke (cerebrovascular diseases): 5.3%
- Accidents (unintentional injuries): 4.8%
- Alzheimer's disease: 3.2%
- Diabetes: 2.8%

- Influenza and Pneumonia: 2.2%

Note that heart disease and cancer kill almost 50% of the total population! Guess what health professionals worldwide cannot deny?

What we eat has an incredible ability to prevent, stop, treat, and/or reverse the onset and development of almost every health condition imaginable!

The point that I'm making is that in order to thrive and live long, you have to incorporate an organized approach to nutrition into your life. There's no way around it. The great news for all of us is that Green Smoothies deliver a stunning amount of unspoiled, miraculous nutrition in every mouth-watering, health-loaded serving! I'll be blunt, drinking Green Smoothies regularly will add years to your life, and make those years far more enjoyable.

Those are just a few more reasons why I am so committed to the Green Smoothie lifestyle. Green Smoothies make everything better for everyone! Remember this:

1. Exercise is very enjoyable!
2. Healthy food intake with Green Smoothies is delicious, simple, and fun!

In order to understand how Green Smoothies can become a daily part of your positive changes in life, we should probably first understand a little more about the history of the human diet. We need to see where we came from (in a dietary sense), where we are, and why. Don't worry - this will be short and sweet!

Chapter 2

Free Radicals and Antioxidants

I promise not to bore you to tears with too much scientific talk throughout this book. There are some key concepts that need to be addressed so that we all can truly appreciate why and how Green Smoothies are so good for us! It really is amazing to consider the nutrient value of a Green Smoothies, especially when you compare it with the nutrient values of so many other commonly consumed food sources.

One of those key concepts involves free radicals and antioxidants. Somehow we all seem to know the two are related, but how? Why are free radicals bad for us and how do antioxidants help to prevent and reverse the damage they cause?

I always knew I needed to understand how free radicals and antioxidants have so much meaning to human health. One day, I just dove in and studied up on the subject! I'm glad I took the time because now I understand how much control I have over my own health. Put simply, antioxidants help to block free radical damage from occurring - and even to neutralize the free radicals altogether! Let's take a closer look:

Free Radicals

Simply defined, free radicals (or just radicals) are unstable, organic molecules. It's widely accepted now that free radicals have a lot to do with cellular damage, the onset of certain diseases – and even aging! Saying that radicals are unstable refers to the fact that they are missing an electron from their atomic structures. They know they're unstable too!

In fact, free radicals travel throughout the body searching for easy molecules to bond with, steal an electron from, and then leave the previously healthy structure in an unstable form. They roam around freely and are able to steal electrons from a wide variety of other structures.

Free radicals are thieves and body wreckers that care only about themselves!

To be fair, radicals do have a couple of positive functions. First, they help phagocytes (white blood cells) consume harmful bacteria and pathogens that live inside the body. In addition, it is believed that free radicals play a key role in the redox signaling process, which transfers cellular messages.

When a free radical steals an electron from a cell wall, that structure is left unstable. It in turn becomes a free radical itself and thus creates a snowball effect of harmful damage throughout the body. Aging may not be altogether preventable, but much of the damage commonly caused by free radicals is. By reducing the number of free radical molecules present in your body at any given time, you are reducing your probability of experiencing an array of different possible types of cellular damage.

This accumulative damage is what adds up to aging!

Free radicals come from environmental pollutants including smoke, herbicides, poisons, and other toxic substances. They form as a natural byproduct of human metabolism. Radicals are all around us most of the time. In the middle of America, it's quite difficult to escape regular exposure to free radical substances. The best thing we humans have for reducing our exposure to them, and thereby reducing our respective probabilities for experiencing their harmful effects, is to blast these radicals with antioxidants!

Antioxidants

Antioxidants are organic molecules found primarily in vegetables and fruits that combat the numerous negative effects of free radicals. More specifically, they are found in the vitamins that our food sources contain, especially Vitamins E, C, A (in beta-carotene form), and selenium. Additionally, antioxidants are found in high doses in natural plant chemical substances, aka phytochemicals.

Antioxidants are like powerful barriers that stop free radicals from causing cellular damage!
Just stick with me a little longer and we'll be through with this technical stuff. Then we can get on to the exciting, mouth-watering part of the book: Green Smoothies!

The Oxidation Process

Oxidation is a process that involves two basic occurrences:

1. Oxygen is added to a substance.
2. Electrons are lost from the substance.

Now, when electrons are lost as a result of oxidation, ionic molecules are created and called free radicals. As we know, free radicals are very detrimental to the body. In general, adding oxygen to a substance begins to break that substance down like an apple's meat turning brown as a result of contact with the air.

Like the apple, the human body breaks down as a result of exposure to free radicals, which are natural byproducts of oxidation.

People create free radicals every time they talk, eat, move, exercise, or even breath! All of these functions, anything and everything we do, produce more free radicals for our systems to face. That's why it's so important to have a very regular delivery schedule when it comes to fresh supplies of antioxidants.
By increasing the antioxidant content of the foods you consume, you will help your body to:
- Enhance immune system effectiveness.
- Reduce the chances of developing cardiovascular disease, various forms of cancer, and more.
- Slow down the aging process.

By increasing your intake of antioxidants, you significantly improve your body's ability to ward off disease and avoid all the other damages that free radicals can cause. As you might expect, fresh foods provide more ready, quality antioxidants than do supplements and other sources. Although antioxidants are available in many food sources, they are especially concentrated in vegetables (especially green, leafy varieties), fruits, nuts, legumes, whole grains, sprouts, and seeds.

It's not surprising that antioxidants appear in high concentration in lip-smacking, ultra-healthful Green Smoothies. By incorporating select antioxidant-rich ingredients in your smoothie recipes, you can stay loaded with them – and thereby, continually thwart the attempts of free radicals to cause any damages to your precious cellular structures!

Green Smoothies deliver loads of life-saving antioxidants, vitamins, fiber, water, minerals, and phytonutrients!

Chapter 3

Why Green Smoothies?

We understand that the importance of nutrition is undeniable. The simple matter is that to live a healthy lifestyle, fight off disease, and increase longevity, we have to embrace the guidelines of proper and helpful food choices. Of course, this book is all about the sheer power and effect of Green Smoothies! So why Green Smoothies? It's because they pack such a nutritional punch that you can't ignore them! Green Smoothies are the Mike Tyson of food power! They are the lions of the food jungle!

8 Fast Green Smoothie Facts

1. Green Smoothies contain large amounts of vitamins and other very beneficial constituents, including minerals, antioxidants, anti-inflammatory, phytonutrients, bioflavonoids, fiber, water, and more!
2. Green Smoothies provide your body with chlorophyll. Chlorophyll is proven to be just one atom different in molecular structure than human blood. Drinking and assimilating the ready goodness of a Green Smoothie is much like receiving a cleansing blood transfusion!

3. When combined with the recommended 60% organic fruit and 40% green leafy vegetable ratio, Green Smoothies are very easy to digest. Follow the proper preparation guidelines (provided later) and blend your smoothies well. Adequate blending homogenizes the nutrients and makes them super-simple to assimilate. In fact, these delicious smoothies are so bio-available that they start to absorb into your system even while still in your mouth!

4. Although fresh-made juices are delicious and nutritious, they are not considered a real food source. That's because they have little or no fiber. Green Smoothies are considered a whole food source because they retain 100% of their natural fiber content.

5. Green Smoothies are totally delicious! Blended with about three to five fresh, organic fruits, Green Smoothies are dominantly sweet, but balanced with earthy, wholesome green leafy vegetable goodness. Children, adults, and even our favorite pets can benefit greatly from Green Smoothies.

6. It's simple to make Green Smoothies – and cleanup is a breeze too! I keep my fruits and greens in separate containers in the fridge. I have them ready to go so that it's always a streamlined process (more on this later). When I'm done blending the smoothie, I just rinse the blender jar, and it's ready for the dishwasher. While the blender is running, I put the different fruit and green containers back in the fridge, and I'm almost finished cleaning up even before the smoothie has finished blending!

7. Any human being that's at least six months old can enjoy the natural strength of Green Smoothies. Babies love the sweet tastes. Toddlers think of them as treats, teenagers love them, men and women alike appreciate the health benefits they pack, as well as the increased vitality they bring into our lives.

8. There are an unlimited number of Green Smoothie possibilities with which to experiment. That means that Green Smoothies are infinitely versatile. There's an always different combination to experiment with, another fruit/vegetable/green combination is just waiting for you to find. Everyone can have a favorite Green Smoothie recipe of their own!

Of course, I could go on and on about numerous other Green Smoothie benefits, but we will discover loads of these as we progress through this book.

In the next sections, we will get into all of the super-healthy ingredients of Green Smoothies. When you learn about all the unspoiled, nutrient-loaded goodness contained in Green Smoothies, you'll completely understand why they are considered by nutritionists and other health professionals worldwide to be the ultimate food source.

Chapter 4

Nutrition of the Green Smoothie

The fact is that many people, billions, in fact, make poor food choices on a daily basis. Now, I don't want to sound heartless. I understand that a large percentage of the world population has little to no choice concerning what they are privileged enough to eat. I'm talking about the rest of the population, those who do have choices about the foods they eat. So many people go through their lives giving no consideration to the enormous amounts of non-nutritious, even toxic, food sources that they take into their bodies.

Remember this: Anything you put into your body has to be broken down, extracted from, absorbed and disposed of by your body.

Fresh, organic Green Smoothies have little to no harmful ingredients. In fact, they are some of the healthiest, most easily absorbed foods ever prepared. Let's take a closer look at just what's included in a Green Smoothie!

Water

It should be no major news flash that water is vitally important to life and health. Second in importance to maintaining life only to the air we breathe, water sustains us, heals us, and enables us to remain vital. Depending on which part of the body you consider, the human body is made up of between 22% and 90% water. For instance, your brain consists of about 90% water. Muscle tissue is made up of roughly 75% water, and our bone material is just about 22% water. Blood is more than 80% pure water. Overall, the human body is roughly two-thirds water.

Green Smoothies are also water-rich, just like our bodies! When you drink Green Smoothies on a daily basis, you increase your hydration – and that's definitely a good thing! Dehydration causes a long list of health issues and water combats all of them in a powerful style. Taking in more water will help your body to:

- Efficiently transport oxygen and nutrients throughout your body
- Think clearly
- Keep the air you breathe moist to keep your lungs functioning well
- Enhance metabolic functioning
- Shield vital organs from harmful substances and organisms
- Regulate its temperature effectively and efficiently
- Keep the liver and blood detoxified

- Keep its joints lubricated
- Plus more

It's true that every cell from the bottom of your feet to the top of your head needs water. Without adequate and regular hydration, things get ugly fast on a cellular level. So, keep blending up those ultra-tasty, water-rich Green Smoothies to keep your cells hydrated and thriving!

Fiber

Fiber is a substance made up of non-digestible plant threads and filaments. Although your body cannot digest fiber, it is nonetheless very important for developing and sustaining optimal health. It has been repetitively proven in clinical studies that diets high in fiber are extra helpful at:

- Maintaining a healthy digestive system
- Controlling blood-glucose levels
- Lowering cholesterol
- Preventing the development of cancerous cells
- Maintaining a healthy weight

Making sure you take in plenty of fiber rich food is an important step toward developing optimal health. It just so happens that Green Smoothies are a natural source of life-enhancing fiber. Yes! Yet another fact about Green Smoothies that make them an undeniably intelligent food choice.

Vitamins

There's always a lot of talk about vitamins. I remember my dad going on a Vitamin kick back in the early 1970s. He gave me Niacin (Vitamin B3, nicotinic acid), and I must have been deficient in it because it made me feel really warm. From then on, I had a fascination with vitamins, although it took me many years afterward to learn all the nuances and differences in and about vitamins. Everyone seems to have an opinion, and that's fine, but as it happens, there are a lot of misconceptions about vitamins too.

Just what are vitamins and what roles do they play in developing and sustaining human health?

Vitamins composition are pretty simply. They are just organic compounds essential for metabolism. To date, thirteen vitamins have been identified. Vitamin-like substances known as bioflavonoids (see phytonutrients) are strongly believed to bring about a vast array of beneficial health advantages. If an organism is deficient in one or more vitamins, it may develop specific disorders, as determined by which vitamin or vitamins is/are deficient. So, it's a good thing that it takes just a tiny bit of vitamins, normally just a milligram or two of each daily to remain in good health.

There are fat-soluble and water-soluble vitamins. Fat-soluble vitamins include A, D, E, and K while the B complex Vitamins and Vitamin C comprise the water-soluble list. Our bodies are capable of storing fat-soluble vitamins in our liver, but water-soluble vitamins are not well stored. For this reason, we need to keep resupplying ourselves with water-soluble vitamins on a regular basis.

Here are just a few things that our body uses vitamins for:

- Healthy, glowing skin, and hair
- Strong bones, teeth, and nails
- Blood clotting ability
- Night vision
- Maintaining muscle tone
- Manufacturing blood cells
- Metabolizing energy
- Normalizing blood-glucose levels
- Synthesizing antibodies
- Healing wounds
- The list goes on and on!

Green leafy vegetables and other delicious, colorful vegetables are the best sources for life-yielding vitamins. Green Smoothies are one of the world's absolute best sources for delivery of unspoiled, raw, organic vitamins, all types of them! Every Green Smoothie you drink is loaded down with all-important vitamins. Your body and brain will be thanking you and thanking you!

Minerals

Minerals are made up of inorganic matter vital to human health and survival. They are neither plants nor animals. It's interesting that minerals are what are formed when you burn plants and animals. Our human bodies are roughly 4% minerals.

There are several categories that minerals are classified into, macro, micro or "trace," and electrolyte. The macro-minerals are so named because they are needed and stored in larger quantities than most other minerals. The macro-minerals include calcium, magnesium, and phosphorous. Micro or trace minerals were more numerous and include:

- Copper
- Manganese
- Chromium
- Fluoride
- Iron
- Molybdenum
- Iodine
- Selenium
- Zinc

Then, there are the three electrolyte minerals: sodium, potassium, and chloride. These three minerals are special because they conduct electrical charges within the body to help accommodate muscle contraction and nerve function. They also keep the body's fluid levels balanced.

We need minerals to perform a variety of functions including:

- Manufacturing hemoglobin
- Developing and maintaining strong bones and teeth
- Protecting cells from oxidative damages
- Synthesizing metabolic enzymes
- Manufacturing digestive juices

When you incorporate daily Green Smoothies into your life, you enter into a zone of internal power that's difficult to beat down. You guessed it – Green Smoothies are also one of this planet's best sources for vitality-enhancing dietary minerals!

Phytochemicals (Phytonutrients)

Phyto is Greek for "plant" and so phytochemicals refer to the natural chemical compounds found in plants. Scientists speculate that there may be as many as 10,000 phytochemicals, many not yet discovered. The phytochemicals may be very beneficial for the prevention, treatment, and reversal of various human health issues, including cancer, metabolic syndrome, stroke, cardiovascular disease, and many more.
The phytochemical nutrients found in Green Smoothies are amazing antioxidants that have the power to annihilate free radicals. There are many different types, including zeaxanthin, kaempferol, tannins, carotene-alpha & beta, lutein, and many others. Each has its strengths, but none has any weaknesses.

By diversifying your Green Smoothie ingredients, you maximize your intake of a variety of life-enhancing phytonutrients!

Thousands of years ago, people figured out that certain elements in certain food sources were very effective at treating their health conditions. If you go back less than 200 years, plant-based medicines were all people had. There were no big pharmaceutical corporations back then. There were no AMA-certified medical doctors pushing the big pharmaceutical products. There were only traditional healers who used medicinal plants to help people feel better, treat disease and maintain health. It wasn't that long ago!

Different phytonutrients provide different health benefits. That's why it's important to diversify your choices between Green Smoothie ingredients. Mix it up folks! When you do, you will be rewarded with a nice medley of fibrous materials, antioxidants, anti-inflammatories, and much more. Just remember that cooking and other forms of manipulating fruits and vegetables diminish the content of nutrients in them. So, consume yours in the whole form.

Although there are various choices available between phytochemical extracts and supplements, it's always best to gain your organic phytochemical nutrients from whole food sources. The raw fruits and green leafy veggies in Green Smoothies provide loads of many different phytonutrients. Of course, constantly munching all those fruits and vegetables takes a lot of time and makes the jaws quite sore. What can be done you ask?

The answer is deliciously obvious: gain daily supplies of wholesome, raw-form phytochemical nutrients by drinking Green Smoothies!

Chapter 5

Greens, Fruits, and Vegetables

One of the things I love most about Green Smoothies is that you never have to drink the same type twice (unless you want to). There are an infinite number of recipes that you can easily create, depending on the types of nutrients you want to include in them. You can blend up an Orange-Strawberry-Baby Spinach Green Smoothie to blast your cells with antioxidant power or even a Cranberry-Asparagus-Kale Green Smoothie to help detoxify your body and blood.

Whatever the case and whatever a person's particular needs, Green Smoothies are an intelligent, economical, and very effective approach to developing and maintaining optimal health levels. Consider the following greens and fruits, as well as hundreds of others readily available whenever you're set to enjoy your next fortifying Green Smoothie!

Before we get into the Green Smoothie recipes, we need to go through some more nutrition education. It's what makes Green Smoothies the amazing food sources they are! After all, this is a book to learn valuable information from – AND have a lot of fun! So, let's get the science out of the way so we can get into blending up some super-powerful, life-saving Green Smoothies.

6 Popular Types of Green Leafy Vegetables with Nutritional Information

Green leafy vegetables are some of the best food sources available to humans. For thousands of years, people have benefitted from their high levels of vitamins, minerals, antioxidants, anti-inflammatories, detoxification agents, carotenoids, flavonoids, and more. That's why Green Smoothies are as incredibly powerful as dietary constituents. When you regularly ingest green leafy vegetables, you give your body what it needs to resist the attacks of oxidation, inflammation, toxification, and much more!

1. Cabbage

Cabbages along with Brussels sprouts, broccoli, and cauliflower, are a member of the cruciferous vegetable family. Although the different types of cabbages are not as nutritious overall as some other family members, they are still loaded with vital nutrients that will make your Green Smoothies healthy, energizing, and naturally tasty!

Cabbage is an excellent source of Vitamin C, a natural antioxidant. It's very low in calories and contains an impressive amount of fiber. Red cabbages have roughly twice the Vitamin C of green cabbages. On the other side of the coin, green cabbages contain roughly twice the folate as do red cabbages. Cabbage is helpful for preventing colon cancer and other malignancies associated with estrogen stimulation.

1 cup of raw green cabbage has:

- 20 calories

- 33 mg of Vitamin C (54% RDA)
- 85% RDA Vitamin K
- Provides a good source of magnesium, calcium, iron, thiamine, phosphorous, potassium, Vitamin B6, and manganese
- Almost no cholesterol
- Almost no fat
- Almost no sodium

2. Chard (Swiss chard)

Swiss chard or just chard is a green leafy vegetable that displays red stalks, leaf veins, and stems. It's known for its sweet beet-like taste and delicate texture. Scientists have discovered that chard has thirteen unique polyphenol antioxidants including kaempferol, syringic acid, and betalains.

I love using Swiss chard in my Green Smoothies, maybe even more than I like spinach!

The phytonutrients in chard, among other functions, help it to live up to its worldwide reputation as a champion antioxidant, blood-glucose stabilizer, anti-inflammatory, and detoxifying agent. In short, Swiss chard is one of the world's best food sources. It's a nutritional powerhouse vegetable that you should enjoy on a regular basis!

Furthermore, just 1 cup of raw Swiss chard contains:
- 715.9% DV of Vitamin K
- 214.3% DV of Vitamin A

- 52.5% DV of Vitamin C
- 37.6% DV of magnesium
- About 30 calories
- A good source of potassium, iron, fiber, copper, calcium, protein, choline, zinc, and more.

3. Collards

A well-known food in the raw food arena, collard greens, are packed full of vitamins, minerals, phytonutrients, and deliciousness like few other foods have been, are, or will ever be. Collards are nutritionally similar to kale but are a heartier, chewier green leafy vegetable. Its taste is on the stronger side than kale. The leaves of collard greens are wide and large.

Collard greens are a superior agent for binding to bile acids throughout the digestive tract. That means that collards are an excellent digestive enhancer, but that's certainly not all! That strong bile acid- binding ability makes collards very effective at lowering cholesterol (which bile acids are synthesized from).

Collard greens are amazingly powerful - and scrumptious!

Additionally, collard greens are gaining a huge reputation as a cancer inhibitor. That's because of their unique combination of four separate glucosinolates: gluconasturtiian, glucotropaeolin, glucoraphanin, and sinigrin. All four can be converted to ITC (isothiocyanates), which kick in detoxification and anti-inflammatory systems, helping to thwart the development of cancer.

1 cup of raw collard greens provides:
- 1045% DV of Vitamin K
- 308.3% DV of Vitamin A
- 57.6% DV of Vitamin C
- More than 40% DV of manganese and folate

- A good source of Omega-3 fatty acids, iron, potassium, phosphorous, Vitamin B6, choline, tryptophan, and more
- 50 calories
- Antioxidant properties
- Anti-inflammatory properties
- Support for cardiovascular health
- Support for efficient digestion
- Lowered cholesterol

4. Kale

Loaded up with many vitamins like K, A, C, and more, Kale is extremely healthy. Kale is notorious for lowering the risks associated with developing prostate, ovary, breast, colon, and bladder cancer – and probably many other types as well! Like collard greens, kale has a nice assortment of ITCs (isothiocyanates) that help the body fight cancer.

Kale contains two highly concentrated and powerful types of antioxidants: flavonoids and carotenoids. There are at least 45 different flavonoids in kale, increasing its value as an effective anti-inflammatory agent.

Kale makes you feel strong and good looking!

Kale provides comprehensive support for the body's detoxification system. New research has shown that the ITCs made from kale's glucosinolates can help regulate bodily detoxification at a genetic level. Its ruffled leaf edges range in color from black to purple to cream and more, all dependent on the variety of kale you select. Kale has an earthy taste that is not overpowering.

Every 1 cup serving of raw kale provides:
- Defense against cancer
- Cardiovascular support
- Lots of fiber
- 1327.6% DV of Vitamin K
- 354.1% DV of Vitamin A
- 88.8% DV of Vitamin C

- A good amount of copper, tryptophan, Vitamin B6, potassium, Omega-3 fatty acids, iron, magnesium, and more
- Just 35 calories

5. Spinach

Perhaps the most beloved green leafy vegetable of all, spinach is one of the planet's super foods for a lot of excellent reasons. To begin with, the vibrantly green leaves of spinach appeal to the eyes and nourish the body in uncountable ways. Spinach is certainly my personal favorite green leafy vegetable! Its dark green color comes from it's carotenoids, including lutein and zeaxanthin, which are known to reduce macular degeneration.

You'll see that I talk A LOT about spinach. I love it! Additionally, more than a dozen flavonoids are present in spinach, making it an excellent anti-inflammatory and anti-cancer agent. Spinach is a stand-alone champion amongst green leafy vegetables in that it is the only one that contains a special group of flavonoids called methylenedioxy flavonol glucuronides. These little nutrients of power have been shown to slow down the cell division in human stomach cancer growths. Calorie for calorie, spinach is famous for being the world's most nutritious food – out of all of them! That's a powerful distinction – and the primary reason why I choose spinach for the majority of my personal Green Smoothie recipes. Mild tasting and unbeatable in nutritional content, spinach is an amazing food source that can lengthen and better your life!

1 cup of raw spinach provides:
- 1110.6% DV of Vitamin K
- 377.3% DV of Vitamin A
- 84% DV of manganese
- 64.7% DV of folate
- Loads of Vitamin C, Vitamin B2, calcium, potassium, iron, fiber, protein, zinc, and so much more
- Anti-inflammatory and anti-cancer benefits
- Cardiovascular benefits
- Almost zero fat and cholesterol
- Very low sodium
- Glycemic load of zero
- Less than 10 calories

6. Turnip Greens

Tasty, stuffed, and filled with all types of beneficial nutrients, turnip greens are difficult to beat as a complete food source. Their slightly bitter taste is a result of their incredible calcium content. Although turnip greens are effective at providing numerous health benefits, they stand out amongst other green leafy vegetables in their ability to fight the development of cancerous cells. This is because turnip greens affect three separate bodily systems simultaneously:

1. The detoxification system
2. The anti-inflammatory system
3. The anti-oxidizing system

Turnip Greens are especially helpful for preventing cancer development. Turnip Greens are also strong supporters of cardiovascular health, digestive efficiency, inflammation reduction, and more. For thousands of years, people all over the planet have cultivated these greens. Turnip greens are super-nutritious, extra delicious, and are an ultra-healthy plant food that will make your Green Smoothies taste robust and deliver optimal vitality!

1 cup of raw turnip greens provides:

- 661.6% DV of Vitamin K
- 219.6% DV of Vitamin A
- 65.7% DV of Vitamin C
- 42.4% DV of folate
- Plenty of manganese, calcium, fiber, copper, Vitamin E, Vitamin B6, potassium, iron, and much more
- Less than 20 calories
- Glycemic load of 1
- No fat, no cholesterol, and very little sodium

So there you have it, six wonderfully healthy green leafy vegetables to include in roughly 40% of every Green Smoothie you blend up! Of course, there are many others too. Consider experimenting with broccoli greens, mustard greens, bok choy, arugula, quinoa, and more. Green leafy vegetables are nearly impossible to beat as overall nutritional food sources and mixing them with fresh organic fruits to make Green Smoothies is a no-brainer for taste, fun, and ultimate health!

Chapter 6
Starting Up

Getting Your Head around the Concept

Being mentally prepared is the key to success. You are going to upend your diet completely and, initially at least, this is going to mean some adjustments.
Let's face it; you are going to be in for some discomfort – no change that is worthwhile is completely painless. That said, the discomfort is not going to be as extreme as it would be if you were fasting – you are still getting all the food groups that you need. For those coffee junkies out there, this will be a little tough but that is why we have included green tea as well.
You can drink up to 3 cups of green tea a day and, because of the caffeine content of the tea, caffeine withdrawal will not be as pronounced. The tea should have no milk in it and should only be sweetened with stevia or a little honey. It is because of the symptoms of Detoxing that I advise starting over a weekend.
By Monday or Tuesday morning you will be feeling a whole lot better – you just need to get through the first weekend. The Epsom salts baths will also help to soothe the aches and pains and to speed up this initial detox period so that will help as well. Any discomfort that you undergo is going to be short-lived. Keep that in mind and you'll get through it.

Smoothies are Complete Meals

We often look at smoothies as a nice side beverage. Consequently, we tend to look at a plan like this one and think that we are going to starve. What we must remember, is that smoothies are a full meal. With this plan, the smoothie recipes have been carefully chosen to provide a balanced meal.You get enough fiber to help you feel full and the nutrients provided will give you a consistent supply of energy without the spikes and crashes that make you feel ravenous.

Selecting and Storing Fruits and Vegetables

Now we have a better understanding of why Green Smoothies are a powerful and concentrated food source. We know how they can help us to live healthier, happier lives, so it's time to get into some delicious, ultimately nutritious Green Smoothie recipes! Of course, I am including some of my personal favorites, but also some that I feel are best for detoxing, best for increased energy, best cancer preventative, and so on.

However, before we get to the actual recipes, let's talk real quick about some common sense guidelines for selecting and storing your vegetables and fruits. While there's nothing fancy to learn, it does help to develop an organized approach to smoothie making. In the long run, these helpful tips will save you time, energy, frustration, and money. When I started making smoothies, I would throw all my produce items in the crisper compartment of my fridge. Every time I would make a smoothie I would prep them, one by one, as needed – and that seemed completely reasonable to me. Then, when I started getting into the smoothie lifestyle, I realized I was spending a lot of time in my kitchen performing repetitive actions like washing, prepping, and cleaning up. Over time, I've developed some simple and effective habits that have streamlined my Green Smoothie operations.

Preparation of Food

Set aside some time to look out for good, healthy fruits and vegetables.Go to your local farmer's market nice and early in the morning to get the best selection of fruits, vegetables, and herbs.It is best to try and get locally grown organic produce. Also, look for products like raw milk, kefir, farm butter, etc.

These fresh products usually taste a lot better than the store bought varieties and are a lot less likely to have chemicals and preservatives. Check to see if there is an organic farm nearby and find out whether or not they deliver vegetable/fruit boxes.Many of the organic farms offer to deliver to your home or office, and they make up a box of the fruits and vegetables that are in season and ready for harvest.Remember that organically grown produce may not look as perfect as the stuff that you find in the stores.

The upside is that it has not been sitting in storage and transferred long distances just to be storage and placed on the grocery store shelves with no idea how long it has been there. The imperfections are a sign that the produce is natural and good for you. When selecting your produce, don't be afraid to try different combinations. You will see in the recipe section, there are a lot of different options – white beans, for example, make a creamier smoothie.

Kefir provides a great source of protein and calcium but also provides valuable probiotics as well. Switching up the base of your smoothie will give you a wider variety of nutrients. It allows you to experiment with different fruits and fats to find the perfect combination of nutrition and flavor for your tastes.

Prepare as Much as Possible

If the morning is a mad rush for you, you might want to consider getting up 15 minutes earlier so that you have a bit more time.

You can, however, also cut back on the time needed to make your smoothies every morning with the following tips:

- *Keep all the necessary ingredients together* – set aside space in the kitchen cupboard to keep all of your smoothie spices, nuts and seeds together.

You can even make little packs with the right amount of nuts, seeds and spices for one smoothie in each.

- *If you want to, you can chop up your fruit and vegetables the night before, put them in an airtight bag and freeze them.*

Freezing your fruits and veggies keeps you from having to put ice in the smoothie and saves time in the morning.

- *When you have to grind seeds, like with flaxseeds, it is best to do that just before you are ready to use them.*

You can, however, measure out how much you need and get it ready in the grinder, or for those of us less technically inclined, in the mortar and pestle.

Plan for the day ahead. Think about what smoothies you are going to want to have the next day and prepare the ingredients the night before. You want to ensure that you do have all the necessary ingredients before you start to prepare your smoothies. The last thing you want to find out when you are getting ready in the morning is that you ran out of your favorite greens!

Tips for Selecting and Storing Green Smoothie Ingredients

1. Keep your produce purchasing decisions diverse by choosing in-season fruits and vegetables? Always be bold and experiment with new fruits and vegetables that you may have never even tried before. Giving your body a wide range of minerals, vitamins, phytonutrients, and other beneficial elements arealways best. In-season produce also is at top quality levels – and offers the best pricing. Remember to support your local organic farmers!

2. Keep track of how much produce you actually use and how much is wasted. Give some realistic thought to how much produce you and your family actually use for the period of time you are shopping for. Remember that fresh produce is best used right away, so don't space your shopping days too far apart.

3. Always inspect fruit and vegetables closely before purchasing. Look for signs of rot, under-ripeness, poor development, bruising, discoloration, malformation, and anything else that may grab a hold of your senses. Also, use your nose! Our noses are one of the best tools we have for determining what we should, or should not, eat.

4. Make sure the produce you choose is at least close to being optimally ripe. Fruits and vegetables are maximally nutritious when properly ripe – and maximizing nutrient levels are what Green Smoothies are all about! You can sometimes buy under-ripe produce and let it finish the ripening process at home. This saves an occasional trip to the grocery.

5. Develop a sincere understanding of just how important it is to choose organic produce whenever possible. Yes, in most cases, organic choices cost a little more. However, be aware of the vast nutritional and other health differences that result when a given fruit or vegetable is NOT repetitively doused in pesticides, herbicides, and other chemical concoctions. Natural plants were not meant to constantly combat all those chemicals. Doing so depletes nutrients, hinders proper development, and poisons the plant.Organic may cost a little more, but isn't your health and wellbeing worth it?

6. Keep produce stored in a cool and dry spot. If you have certain fruits or vegetables that are ripening too quickly, place those in the refrigerator. Remember that many produce items can be frozen, if needed and then used later. When making Green Smoothies, frozen ingredients add coldness and fun!

7. When some produce items are difficult to find, you can add diversity to your Green Smoothies by choosing 100% juices. It's best, of course, to use fresh, whole produce in your smoothies. However, in a pinch, 100% pure cranberry, pomegranate, cherry, carrot, blueberry, or other type of juice works out just fine. It's not always possible to get certain desired fruits and vegetables at your local market, but you can normally find a nice selection of available juices.

A special tip for storing Green Smoothie produce ingredients.

Here's one of my favorites: Using seal-tight plastic storage containers. I normally shop for produce twice each week. Shopping twice a week keeps me loaded up with Green Smoothie ingredients without having my fridge overstuffed and unmanageable. It also reduces spoiled food and waste.

When I get home from the grocery, I clean all the fruits and vegetables that I'll be using for the next three or four days. Then, leaving them in whole form whenever possible, I place each separate type of produce in appropriately sized plastic storage containers – you know, like the Glad or Zip-Lock type. These containers are affordable versatile, stackable, and very easy to use. **Note that some cheap off-brand containers available at some dollar stores are not worth messing with! They are poorly made, don't seal properly, and should not be used. Go for the name brands on these. It will save you money, effort, and frustration in the long run.**

Now, with my produce washed, sorted, and placed in storage containers, I can simply put them in the fridge, all stacked nice and neat. They are readily available when it's smoothie-making time. That's when I just grab what I need for the smoothie at hand. I use the fresh, clean produce inside and then rinse the empty containers in the sink. Then, after a quick rinse of the blender, I'm done! From beginning to end, the Green Smoothie making process takes me only about five or six minutes, clean up included. Then, I'm walking away from a clean kitchen, nutrient-loaded Green Smoothie in hand. Oh yeah!

Keeping your fruits and vegetables clean, fresh, and ready will maximize your smoothie-making enjoyment while minimizing the work involved. After a while, you'll naturally develop your own short cuts. It becomes easier to determine just the right amounts of produce to buy at the store. In no time at all, you'll be a Green Smoothie Master – able to run the whole show with smoothness, efficiency – and much betterhealth and deliciousness in hand!

Chapter 7

Benefits of Green Smoothies

The "smoothie" diet is becoming a rage around the world. People from all walks of life seem to be adopting this "greener" way of life. It is being discussed and debated by people across all echelons of society. The proponents of the green smoothie diet are manycelebrities on TV, athletes, businesspeople, your neighbor across the road. Have you ever wondered what makes the green diet so popular? Undeniably, this diet brings with it a host of benefits. People who have tried this diet once swear by it. Let us explore the benefits of choosing a green smoothie diet.

Easy to prepare

All you need for making your sumptuous smoothie is a blender and some fruits and vegetables. Smoothies can be whipped up in a jiffy and needs no preparation time. It fits into your busy schedule.

Fruits and veggies for your body

The smoothie diet will ensure that you get your recommended dose of fruits and vegetables every day. Eating fruits and vegetables every day is a chore for most people. Green smoothies are easy to consume, so your body gets the fruit and vegetables that it needs.

Easy to digest

Food in a "smoothie" form is gentle on the stomach and easy to digest. Besides, they give you the dietary fiber that you require. You will not experience indigestion or constipation while on a smoothie diet.

Healthy weight loss program

Your smoothie diet is a healthier way to lose weight. You do not need to starve yourself, and your body gets all the nutrition that it requires. You can choose ingredients that aid weight loss and make healthy smoothies that make you lose weight the natural way.
Fortify your immune system
The greens and fruits in your smoothie contain anti-oxidants that help to strengthen your immune system. You are less likely to get sick while on a smoothie diet. Smoothies also have disease-fighting properties.

Build muscles

Green smoothies provide you foods that build your lean mass. The nutrients in a smoothie are easier to digest and it serves your body's requirement without adding any fat. It helps athletes and sportspersons to perform better.

Detoxifies your body

Certain greens like kale and dandelion detoxify the body and neutralize the effect of harmful chemicals that are found all around you. Going on a green smoothie diet may work out to be the best detox program for your body.

Makes you more beautiful/handsome

The vitamins and minerals contained in fruits and veggies take care of your skin, nails and hair. It can give your skin a healthy glow and give your hair that extra bounce. You look and feel better with a smoothie diet.

Energy Boosters

Smoothie diets contain ingredients that can be quickly broken down in the body to give you a surge of energy. These diets energize you to take on the tasks at hand with enhances vigor and enthusiasm.

Better Sleep

Smoothie diets help to regulate your sleep pattern and ensure that you sleep better at night.

Brain food

Smoothie diet gives your brain all the nutrients it needs and helps you to think clearly and with more focus. It can boost your memory too.

Flexi meals

Green smoothies are great at any time of the day. The can replace your main meal or be a healthy snack between meals. You can grab a smoothie anytime you want.

Delicious and irresistible

Smoothies taste great while being healthy. You can easily stick to your smoothie diet since it gives you many options from which to choose. Some of the smoothies are indeed hard to resist.

Healthier than Juices

When you juice a fruit or vegetable, most of the fiber is lost. In smoothies, we use whole fruits and greens. Smoothies take care of the dietary fiber requirements of your body. You might ask why can't I just use fruit juice from the store? Most of the juices that you buy off the shelf contain added sugar and preservatives, which are not good for your body.

Keeps you hydrated

All of us are aware that we need to drink eight glasses of water in a day to keep ourselves hydrated. However, how many of us actually drink the recommended amount of water every day? A smoothie diet ensures that your body gets the required amount of water every day. You just add more water to your smoothies to reach the recommended amount.

Nutrient Boost

Green smoothies traditionally are made with wholesome fruits and vegetables that are high in vitamins, minerals, and other nutrients. After being blended, those ingredients will be in a concentrated form.

Dietary Fiber

Smoothies made with fresh fruits and vegetables are high in dietary fiber that is essential for a number of bodily functions including healthy digestion.

Extra Energy

As an alternative to sugary sodas or caffeine-loaded coffee drinks, try a refreshing green smoothie for an all-natural energy boost.

Holistic Health

Green smoothies can provide a number of health benefits including reduced inflammation, improved digestion, blood purification and even body detoxification.

Weight Loss

Though drinking green smoothies alone won't cause you to lose weight, green smoothies can be part of a healthy diet paired with regular exercise to lose weight. Green smoothies are a great way to fuel your body with necessary nutrients while keeping your calorie count low.

Lasting Energy

While an energy drink might give you a kick of energy for a few hours, you are likely to experience a crash later. Green smoothies, however, have balanced sugar content that helps fuel your body longer.

Cheap and Convenient

Not only are green smoothies incredibly easy to prepare, they are also very inexpensive. You can easily buy produce in bulk, so you always have your favorite smoothie ingredients on hand.

Glowing Skin

The nutrients in green smoothies provide numerous benefits for your skin including clearing up acne and softening your skin.

Shinier Hair

Green smoothies provide you with nutrients and essential oils that your hair needs to stay soft and silky. Drinking green smoothies on a regular basis may also help your hair grow faster.

Antioxidants

Because you are making your smoothie from fresh fruits and vegetables, green smoothies are a great source of antioxidants and phytochemicals. Both help to strengthen your immune system to keep your body healthy.

Chapter 8

Weight Loss Diets and Green Smoothies

Whatever weight loss diet you are following; unlimited amounts of vegetables are probably recommended. But how do you prepare these unlimited amounts of vegetables?

Let's say you get one tablespoon of butter to place on a large serving of cooked vegetables, is the taste satisfying? It is the same problem when you sprinkle a huge salad with a small amount of olive oil. As for the lighter dressings that are commercially available, they often contain additives with unpronounceable names and are packed with sugar!

With green smoothies, you can combine flavors that you like without adding a lot of fats and still feel satisfied.

Speed Up Your Weight Loss

Water Please

You should be drinking at least eight glasses of water a day. That's 2 liters. Drinking enough water is even more vital when you are detoxifying. Getting enough water will help you to deal with the symptoms of detox more effectively. Dehydration during detox is common and can lead to headaches and fatigue. Don't put yourself at risk to feel bad.

The easiest way to ensure that you get enough is to have a bottle on hand with you at all times.If you see the bottle on the desk, it will remind you to drink the water. Remember, you will need to drink 2 liters a day so measure how much water your bottle contains to figure out how many bottles you need to drink a day. And no, tea and coffee and smoothies do not count towards the total in this instance. Avoid commercial flavored waters and water flavoring drops– they tend to have a ton of sugar and chemicals in them.

Drink your water!

It doesn't matter if you do not feel thirsty – if you wait until you feel thirsty, it means that you have already started to dehydrate.

If you are not drinking enough water, the body retains the water it has. Water retention will make it harder to flush the toxins out of your body.

The big benefit of drinking more water – you will find that you no longer feel as hungry – what we often feel as hunger pangs are actually a sign that we are dehydrated.

Drink a glass of water if you are feeling hungry and it might just go away.

Goodnight Sweetheart

Are you one of those people that hits the snooze button over and over again or do you spring out of bed in the morning ready for the day?If you need to keep hitting the snooze button, there is a good chance that you are not getting enough sleep.When you do not get enough sleep, your body is under stress and produces more cortisol. Cortisol in turn suppresses the hormones that control hunger, and you end up eating more calories throughout the day.

The cure for not getting enough sleep is not hard – you simply need to get more. You can rationalize burning the candle at both ends as much as you want, but there is no substitute for getting a full night's sleep.

You will feel more rested and be able to accomplish more after a proper night's rest. You owe it to yourself to make getting enough sleep a priority.

You need to ensure that you get up at the same time every day, regardless of when you went to bed.

Work out the optimal time for you to wake up – you should be up and about at least an hour before you need to leave for work.

Now work out your bedtime – it should be at least 8 hours before you need to get up. Give yourself about 15 minutes to fall asleep.

Give yourself about an hour before bedtime to wind down and relax so that your body starts to prepare for sleep. To do this, you should switch off the TV, your computer, and your tablets and do something that will not stimulate your mind too much in the interim.

In the morning, climb out of bed and open the curtains immediately. According to findings published in Women's Health Magazine, the simple act increasing the amount of exposure to early morning light will decrease the risk of being overweight.

It's not that hard once you get used to it. Try this experiment – pretend that there is a power blackout and don't switch on any lights, etc. for one night. Use candles instead. You'll be amazed at how early you start to become tired. It just goes to show how much artificial light stimulates the mind.

If you are doing the smoothie cleanse, your 7-8 hours of sleep a day becomes even more vital – your body needs the time to really repair and to clear out all the toxins. You will also find, especially during the first few days, that you are going to be more tired.

If you battle to fall asleep at night, you can try the following:

- Keep a notepad and pen next to the bed – if anything is worrying you, write it down and you can deal with it in the morning.

- Add lettuce to your evening smoothie – lettuce induces calm and has a soporific effect.

- Practice good sleep hygiene – block out as much light as possible, block out as much noise as possible and try to keep the room at an even, cool temperature.

Warm Water and Lemon Juice

Now, that you are up, have a glass of tepid water with lemon juice in it.It is best to use fresh lemon juice in your drink. Use freshly squeezed lemons for more a more nutritious beverage. If you use bottled juice, you are adding preservatives, and it does not taste as good as fresh lemon juice. Use the juice of either a half or whole lemon in a whole glass of water.

Lemon water taken in this way will stimulate the detox process, help with digestion, boost immunity, help clear out uric acid, stimulate the mind, reduce inflammation and start the body burning fat. This drink also gives you a dose of Vitamin C.

The question is not so much why you should adopt this habit, but why haven't you already?

Stretch

You know how to stretch; just do it.

Your body loves stretching. If you want, learn a few yoga postures that will help. It really doesn't matter as long as you are elongating the muscles.

Stretching for as little as 5 minutes every morning will help to tone and smooth the muscles in your body; boost circulation and lymph drainage and help you to feel calmer and more relaxed.

Now Move!

I did say that there was no intense exercise program here. There is, however, some exercise.

Every morning, before your morning smoothie, you need to do around 15-30 minutes of cardio. You could walk, cycle, jog – whatever you want, and are able, to do.

If you are a bit of a couch potato, start off slowly.Walk for 5 minutes or 10 minutes.Build it up as you go along. By the end of the nine days, you'll find that you look forward to your exercise time.Even a five-minute walk helps to boost energy levels and gets the heart pumping.

It will help to reduce feelings of anxiety, depression and stress. It will also help you deal with the symptoms of detox. Moving is what the body was designed to do. Get moving, even if it is just a little.Best of all, it speeds up the weight loss benefit of this plan.

You do not need to kill yourself exercising – even walking around the block a few times will be beneficial.If you like these tips so far, *you must* check out my 97 weight loss tips that are available to you

Put Your Back into It

Strength training is another vital component here –
again, you need not kill yourself but do incorporate
some strength training at least every second day.You
don't even have to buy special exercise equipment –
look in your grocery cupboards at home if you're
desperate – a can of baked beans can double as a
dumbbell, at least, initially.

Get creative and you'll soon find that there are plenty
of "weights" that you can use in your home. Strength
training is going to be the key to losing the maximum
amount of weight possible because it will help you to
turn that flab into muscles.

The reason that you are not able to maintain the weight
lost during one of those fad diets, (Remember the
Cabbage Soup Diets?), is your body is starving for
nutrients. When this happens, your body starts to use
muscle mass for energy, not fat. You may lose some
weight initially, but you also lose muscle mass.

And muscle mass is essential for anyone trying to lose
weight – even when the muscle is at rest, it still burns
more energy than fat does.

More muscle = Better fat-burning potential.

That also translates into better energy all the time.

Extra Nutrients

You will also need to take a multi-vitamin every morning.While this plan is going to improvedrastically the nutritional content of your diet, it is still going to be difficult to get all the vitamins and minerals that you optimally need.

Studies have found that those who are deficient in nutrients are more at risk of being overweight, so it is better to ensure that you have enough.You are more likely to overeat if your body is nutrient deficient. You do NOT need to take mega-doses. A simple multi-vitamin supplement will do.

In addition, unless you are eating oily fish twice a week, you are going to need to take a fish oil supplement. And, yes, it has to be fish oil – our bodies are not able to process the Omega-3s in plants.Omega-3s are essential to the body – that is why they are called essential fatty acids. The body uses fatty acids for a range of processes, but the most important benefit is that they reduce inflammation.

Omega-3's can help to protect us from developing depression, heart disease, high LDL cholesterol, degenerative conditions like arthritis and dementia.It also changes the way in which the body uses its fat stores. Omega-3's encourages the burning of fats and triglycerides and prevents the body from storing the visceral fat (belly fat) that is so dangerous in terms of health.

There is one more supplement that may be necessary if you are not going to use yogurt or kefir – a probiotic supplement.Studies have linked visceral fat – the fat stored around the abdomen with decreased levels of the healthy bacteria in the gut. The aim here is to re-populate your gut with healthy bacteria.

Get Family and Friends Involved

It will be important to explain the plan to family and friends so that they can support you.Eating out in social settings is going to be difficult to accomplish and your friends and family need to know what is going on. Be prepared for all the "good" advice and also be prepared for some negative statements. There has been a lot of misinformation spread about smoothies in the past, and a lot of people still think that smoothies are fattening. This eating plan uses real results as it's building blocks and is healthy. What gave smoothies a bad rap was that people were piling in the fruit, etc. and adding in too much sugar, without enough protein.

I once saw a recipe for a smoothie that was essentially just banana and condensed milk mixed in with water. It was practically pure sugar but was being billed as a healthy fruit smoothie. The idea that smoothies are bad for you comes from outdated science and theories. We now know that it is the effect of the food on our blood sugar that is more important than the actual amount of calories or fat that the food contains.

As recently as 15 years ago, we were told that we must stick to a low-fat diet but that sugar was okay because it contained no fat. This information has been disproved, but attitudes, in general, take longer than that to adjust. Let your family know that you are not going to be yourself for the first few days and enlist their support with things like the household chores and cooking and cleaning. You can also mention the fact that you are on this eating plan to colleagues at work if you want to.

It is important to have a good support structure in place when changing the way you do things as a rule. Someone to talk to when it seems easier to break the rules is a very important part of making this work. Choose someone that will offer real support though and not try to force their views on healthy eating onto you as well.

Your New Bath Time Ritual

For the first three nights, you are going to support the detox process by having an Epsom salt bath. After the first week, you can reduce that to two days a week. *Warning: If you suffer from high blood pressure, leave this section out completely.*

You have no doubt seen advertisements for Magnesium oils and sprays that allow you to get your daily dose of Magnesium through the skin. Science has proven that Magnesium can be absorbed efficiently through the skin or taken from the diet. You are now going to benefit from that knowledge, without paying the hefty price tag for the fancy magnesium oils and sprays.

All you need is good old-fashioned Epsom salts. Epsom Salts are made up of Magnesium and Sulfate. All you need to do to get the benefit is to put about two cups of Epsom salts in the bathtub and add hot water. Soak for at least 15 minutes. Keep a big glass of water next to the bath and sip frequently. The water should be at room temperature and should not have any ice in it. I have an Epsom Salt bath two to three times a week – I soak for at least half an hour.

I take a good book with me, and I find that it is very relaxing. Find some way for you to relax in the bath – maybe this means reading a book or magazine or simply lying back listening to music. Do whatever will work for you in this instance. I also add:

- 5-6 drops Juniper essential oil
- 5-6 drops Eucalyptus essential oil
- 5-6 drops Sweet Orange essential oil

The oils are not essential, but they do help to increase the benefits of the bath.

Juniper is good for promoting circulation; Eucalyptus for easing aching muscles and Sweet Orange is good for pepping you up.

I chose these oils because they do not interfere with me sleeping. They help you feel refreshed but not over-stimulated.

Give yourself a vigorous rubdown with your towel afterward to further the effects.

Do this at least an hour before bed to promote better sleep.

Do have a warm blanket on your bed – at first, your body temperature will be raised, but will soon lower again.

You must NOT consume the salts internally.

Unless you are under the supervision of a properly licensed and qualified health care practitioner, it is a really bad idea to consume the salts internally. If ingested they can have a profound laxative effect.

If you have very sore muscles, you can also make a paste of Epsom salts and apply where needed. Mix the salts with enough water to make a stiff paste and apply to the sore area, leave for at least 20 minutes before rinsing off. Do not do this if the skin is broken – it will burn a lot.

Don't apply any lotions or creams of any sort to the skin after this bath. The body needs to sweat to get rid of the toxins and creams will end up getting in the way and clogging the pores.

Chapter 9

What is a Smoothie Cleanse?

One of the most popular diets of the current decade is the smoothie cleanse. The smoothie cleanse, has become extremely popular, due to its simplicity and the level of results that most people can achieve with it. Many people not only decrease their weight but also improve their bodies in a variety of other ways. For example, you may be able to improve your skin clarity, your overall health and even the strength of your hair and bones. And all of that just by eating some smoothies as part of your normal diet.

So what is the smoothie cleanse really? Well, it's a way that you can make your body healthier as well as losing weight. For this cleanse to work you would simply replace some of your snacks and meals with smoothies. Doing so will help you eat less, stay full longer and also clean out a lot of the toxins that enter into your body throughout your normal day as well as throughout your normal eating habits. If you follow a good cleanse you'll start feeling better all-around very quickly.

You start feeling great so quickly with a smoothie cleanse because you are cleaning out your body. The toxins we've talked about are pretty normal for just about everyone. In fact, you'd be hard pressed to find someone who doesn't have these toxins that haven't just completed a cleanse or a detox of some type. That's because we all ingest these toxins without even realizing it, and since we don't realize we've done it, most people don't think about doing anything about it either. After all, why would we fix something that isn't broken?

The reason you start feeling so great so quickly with a smoothie cleanse is because you are actually cleaning out your body. The toxins we've talked about are pretty normal for just about everyone. In fact, you'd be hard pressed to find someone who doesn't have these toxins that hasn't just completed a cleanse or a detox of some type. That's because we all ingest these toxins without even realizing it and, since we don't realize we've done it, most people don't think about doing anything about it either. After all, why would we fix something that isn't broken?

When you cleanse out your body, it removes all of the toxins that got in there without you even realizing it. What happens then is your organs are able to work even better and they're capable of carrying out functions that had been slowed down by all the toxins in your body. The worse the toxin levels are in your body the worse the trouble you're going to experience. You want to make sure that you're paying attention to your body and recognizing when it starts to slow down or when you just don't feel right. These are signs that something is definitely wrong.

The smoothie cleanse process is a way of cleaning out the toxins in a healthy and natural way. When you switch to smoothies, you are removing the unhealthy foods that you would normally reach for when you are hungry. Now instead of digesting unhealthy processed foods full of additives, you will be filling your body with wholesome whole fruits and vegetables, no added preservatives. You will notice a difference once your body is free of additives and toxins, and if you start eating them again, your body will let you know as your prior symptoms start to return.

What you need to do is drink plenty of healthy smoothies. Of course not every smoothie is actually healthy for you. You need to consider the foods and ingredients you are putting into your smoothie in order to get good benefits without just adding a lot of sugar (which is definitely a toxin to avoid). The smoothies that we've included are from a variety of different categories. We've included some that are going to help with the initial detoxification process and some that are going to be good and very healthy to continue using even after your detox. We've also included some that just taste good (and aren't *too* bad for you). You can use those as treats or special snacks.

This section on the smoothie cleanse is going to help you understand how to get started. It's also going to walk you through some of the best smoothie recipes that you can use to get yourself healthier much faster. There is actually a variety of different types of smoothies that you can try including those with fruit, vegetables, high protein and more. So whether you're just looking to lose a little weight, or you're looking to get your entire body healthier you'll be able to.

Chapter 10

How Does the Smoothie Cleanse Work?

A smoothie cleanse works by cleaning out every one of your major organs including the kidneys, tissues and joints. You'll also be able to clean out your bowels, digestive tract, colon, and intestines. All of these aspects of your body are important to your overall health and if you aren't careful to take care of them you're going to experience a lot more health problems than you may have thought. And some of those problems will seem like they came out of nowhere because you don't realize you're doing anything wrong. When you make a smoothie for your smoothie cleanse, you need to focus on a few important aspects. For one thing, you need to think about foods that are good for your body. You need to make sure that you are performing a cleanse somewhat frequently, especially if you're not going to stick to this smoothie diet full-time (which most people won't). When you transition back to eating different foods, you will be returning the toxins that come from processed and chemically treated foods. These toxins will return to your body, and you will need to clean them out again.

Your smoothie needs to include some foods and ingredients that are going to improve your overall health and allow you to do just that. Remember that different ingredients are going to help you in different ways. That's why it's important to include a variety of different ingredients in each smoothie that you prepare so you're targeting a few different areas of the body. Detoxing your body will take a few days to a week. Once you're able to detox your body fully, you can start focusing on getting healthy and losing weight.

The smoothie cleanse works because of the different ingredients used to target different areas including your kidneys, blood, colon and more. When these ingredients are processed by the body they go to work directly with these different areas and help to push the toxins through them and out. It's similar to pushing a plunger into a full container. Whatever is in the container will have to force its way out somehow and when you're done the container will be almost entirely clean. That's what happens with your internal organs. The smoothie cleanse isn't just about getting the toxins out after all. It's actually about making yourself healthier and ensuring that you are staying healthier. You can do this by continuing to add smoothies to your diet and making sure that they are still healthy enough to improve your overall body. This happens by following some of the healthy smoothie recipes that we're going to talk about in the later sections of this book. It's all about fruits, veggies and greens.

Chapter 11

The Best Things to Include in Your Smoothie Cleanse

Now you can put just about anything you want into a smoothie but that doesn't mean it's going to be healthy for you. It also means that you're not going to get the detox benefits that you want. You need to make sure that you're including some of the healthiest ingredients available. We're looking at only natural ingredients because you want to make sure you're getting healthy. To do so you need to avoid a lot of extra fillers, sugar, carbs or anything else that's going to make you put on weight a lot faster than you did before. The point is to get healthy after all.

Some of the best ingredients for your smoothie cleanse we list below. Sure we included some great recipes for you as well but we also understand that you might want to create your own smoothies. If you know which ingredients to use and what benefits they will have in your smoothie, you'll be better prepared to create your own. Plus you'll know why we include some of these great fruits, vegetables and greens in a lot of our recipes and some of them in only a few. We want you to get the best possible benefits so; we combine the best ingredients.

Spinach & Kale – These greens are actually amazing for your colon. Spinach and kale have a lot of fiber, amino acids, calcium, vitamin K, iron, manganese, zinc, and vitamin A. and folate. Each of these vitamins and minerals can do things like improve your skin, improve your immune system and provide antioxidants to your body.

Pears– These fruits are great for the colon as well, but they're also great for your lungs and your skin. This is because they contain a variety of different vitamins (B, C, E& K) as well as copper, manganese, potassium, iron, calcium and zinc. All together these will help you look and feel better.

Lemon– This fruit will work great for detoxification. That's because it contains high levels of alkaline as well as vitamin C, calcium, potassium, and magnesium. Each of these different minerals and vitamins will also help improve your skin, fight out wrinkles, get rid of bacteria, improve liver function get rid of toxins and free radicals and even more. It even helps you to lose more weight.

Cucumber – Great for its anti-inflammatory abilities, cucumbers also help to reduce bloating and improve your skin's clarity and brightness. These anti-inflammatory abilities are because of all the B vitamins, electrolytes, vitamin C, and caffeic acid that are present in these veggies.

Celery – Once again containing high amounts of alkaline, celery also includes calcium, magnesium, potassium, B vitamins, C vitamins, iron, amino acids, polyacetylene and phthalide compounds. Each of these reduces blood pressure and puffiness throughout the body as well as decreasing inflammation, detoxifying your entire body and cleaning out the colon.

Banana– When you're doing a smoothie cleanse you definitely want to make sure your digestive system is working properly because that's what will get rid of those toxins. Bananas include high fiber, vitamin C, potassium, vitamin A and vitamin B6 which will all improve your blood pressure and cholesterol levels as well as improving digestion and reducing constipation.

Cinnamon – This spice will actually help you get rid of bacteria in your body as well as reducing levels of inflammation and contributing antioxidants. Cinnamon has been shown to reduced blood sugar levels in testing, so you stay healthier by using this spice. Even more it's going to improve your brain strength and health to make you even smarter.

Avocado– This is actually a great fruit that helps you to get a lot of nutrients in a very small quantity. They contain high amounts of vitamins B5, B6, C, E, and K as well as folate and potassium. So you get a lot of heart benefits as well as better weight loss, lower blood sugar and lower risk of most diseases including high cholesterol.

Parsley – This is a herb that aids in your digestion and will work excellent for the purpose of your smoothie cleanse because it also flushes out the kidneys and the blood. This great herb will also detoxify your entire body. All of these great benefits come for the vitamins A, C & E as well as iron and antioxidants in the herb itself.

Mint – The final herb we have to look atis mint. Mint contains high amounts of vitamin C and A as well as copper, iron, potassium and calcium. It's great for improving your digestion that will allow you to get rid of more toxins faster.

The more of these ingredients that you include in your smoothie, the better you're going to be able to get rid of the toxins and the better you're going to feel. You want to make sure that you balance them out well as each one has its own distinct flavor and can influence the flavor of your smoothie. As long as you get a little of each of the flavors in though you'll be able to get the distinct benefits that each one has (though to differing degrees of effectiveness).

Chapter 12

Starting Out with the Smoothie Cleanse (The First Few Days)

The first few days of your smoothie cleanse aren't going to be easy. The challenge isn't because of the smoothies themselves, but because you're just not used to this type of diet. You may find yourself a little bit hungry when you first start out, or you may experience problems where you don't like some of the smoothies. If this happens then just try to finish that particular smoothie and don't be too worried about trying a different smoothie when it's time for your next meal. No one is going to expect you to like every smoothie that you try.

Some of the smoothie recipes that we have and that you'll find in other places as well are going to seem a little strange to you. They will mix a variety of different things that you've probably never thought of mixing before. But you don't have to be too worried. The recipes provided are going to help you be healthier than you are now, they are also going to contain differing levels of each ingredient changing their nutritional properties. The purpose of this is for one, so you get the right level or nutrients, and you get the benefits you are targeting. The other reason is so that the flavors don't try to compete with one another and give you a weird taste.

Of course, just like with anything else there will be ingredients or flavors that you don't like. It happens throughout life, and it's something that isn't avoidable. So you want to make sure that you're trying several different options and selecting the ones that work best for your needs or your taste buds. Don't be afraid to experiment on your own either. As you get used to this diet, even more you'll be able to add your own ingredients and still keep the diet healthier than your regular foods.

For the first few days, you'll want to focus on only a small amount of change. This is because changing your entire diet dramatically all at once is never good for anyone. If you try to jump right into this diet with both feet and replace your meals and snacks entirely with smoothies, thinking you're going to get healthier, you're most likely going to fail. It's unfortunate, but this is very true of most people who go on a diet. They start out with the best of intentions but then they end up struggling to keep themselves afloat.

The reason so many people fail right off the bat is because they try to go too far, too quickly. We don't want this to happen to you which is why we're going to walk you through the steps a little slower. The faster you try to jump in, the harder it's going to be. Changing your diet is difficult enough without trying to do a complete 180 on day one. By taking changes slowly, you'll be able to make all the changes you need at a much more successful pace. Making slow changes are important so you can have a much better possibility for success and long term changes.

Because we want you to succeed, we are going to show you step by step how to start. We're going to start you off by only replacing one meal per day with a healthy smoothie. Start by taking your regular breakfast off the menu and replace it with one green or vegetable smoothie instead. Replacing your breakfast is going to get you off to a great start for the day. You'll get plenty of vitamins and minerals as well as a good amount of protein but not a lot of sugar (which is in most fruit smoothies).

At this point, you're still going to eat a regular lunch and a regular dinner that will keep you healthier and help you stave off hunger. You want to make sure that your regular meals are still healthy. Meals should include plenty of fruit and vegetables as well as healthy proteins. Try to stay away from a lot of sugar and starchy foods which could counteract a lot of the benefits you're experiencing with your smoothie.

You're also allowed to eat a couple snacks each day but keep them healthy snacks. Try to avoid junk food as much as possible.

During your initial few days, you should also make sure that you're drinking only water and tea. These beverages do not include sugar or any additives which make them all natural and extremely healthy. They will help you to clean out your system much faster because you're getting all the fluids that your body desperately needs. Not only that, you won't be replacing all the calories that you just got rid of by replacing your breakfast with a smoothie. Juices (even natural fruit juices) and caffeinated beverages are not good for you, and they're going to cause you a lot of trouble in the long run.

Water and tea are quite healthy for you because the primary ingredient even in tea is just water. You're not getting any additives, and you're getting liquid. What you want to do, is drink as much water or tea as possible. Drinking a lot is going to make you feel less hungry, and it's also going to increase the amount of toxins flushed from your body within a very short amount of time. Toxin removal is important to your overall health and the speed at which your cleanse is going to work effectively.

If you can drink a gallon of water per day, you'll be able to reduce your food intake significantly. This is because your body reacts the same way when you're feeling thirsty or dehydrated as it does when you're hungry. So you end up eating when your body didn't want food in the first place. By drinking all that water, you are also going to rehydrate your body that is important when you're detoxifying because you're getting rid of a lot of wastes during this time. It's important to refresh your body consistently, so you don't end up sick from this process.

These instructions are going to get you through the first three days of your diet. If you want to get the best benefits you might want to pick the beginning of a week whether that's a Monday or a Sunday for you to start. Starting at the beginning of the week is going to help you stay on track much better than at the end when you are already tired. It's going to allow you to feel better about yourself. So for the first three days try to stick to at least one smoothie replacement per day. You can select any of the protein or vegetable smoothies we've listed below, and you'll have plenty of options for your entire diet.

Chapter 13

The Benefits of Smoothie Cleansing as a Process of Detoxification

There are many detox diet programs that are popular today, and all of them have one thing in common – they all promote eating fresh and organic fruits and vegetables to flush out the toxins in the body.

Unlike other diets that can make a person starve, the Smoothie Detox diet can make you full and satiated. Even though this eating program is plant based, it allows the incorporation of meat and fish to the diet. It can cleanse the body without depriving it of the essential vitamins and minerals that it needs.

Unlike other diets which can make a person starve, the Smoothie detox diet can make him full and satiated. Even though this eating program is plant based, it allows the incorporation of meat and fish to the diet. It can cleanse the body without depriving it of the essential vitamins and minerals that it needs.

The Smoothie Diet is very friendly, and can be done by anybody. It is ideal for a long-term diet plan. Since the diet is all about eating healthy, it is very safe, and it does not have any drawback.

Here are the ingredients to avoid:

Dairy products - Milk and cream should not be added to the smoothie because they contain extra calories. Plain Greek yogurt is acceptable because it is low in calorie.

Sugar and any other artificial sweetener - If possible, use stevia to sweeten your smoothie because it has no calories. Other natural sweeteners like maple syrup and honey should be used moderately. Too much sweetness from fruits should also be avoided. Although fruits are good for the body, too much could also mean too much sugar. The high amount of sugar in fruit could lead to weight gain.

Chapter 14

The End of Your Smoothie Cleanse

For the second half of your smoothie cleanse you want to make sure that you're eating primarily smoothies for your diet. Now not everyone can switch over to a full smoothie diet, and that's okay. You want to make sure that you're getting the most health benefits as you can from your smoothies. At the same time, you don't want to make yourself sick or starve yourself which can happen if you try to cut your calorie intake too dramatically.

If you can, try to replace all three of your regular meals with smoothies. Make sure you're eating primarily protein, veggie and green smoothies and that you're including fruit smoothies only sporadically as a little treat. If you eat too many of these fruit smoothies, you're going to end up gaining more weight, and you'll have a lot more sugar than you probably did before. By eating only the smoothies and interspersing them with snacks, you will be able to get rid of any toxins in your body within a short period. You'll also be able to get rid of excess weight very quickly too.

When you replace your meals with a smoothie, you're going to be getting fewer calories, fewer carbs, and less fat. Additionally, you will be getting less sugar than you do in eating regular meals. This is especially true if you're one of those people that likes to go out to eat. You will still drink as much water or tea as you can, and you still want to make sure that the snacks you eat consist of fruit, vegetables, nuts or other healthy products. If you eat a lot of sweets or junk food for snacks, you will counteract the benefits of the smoothies, and you'll start adding all those toxins back in, which means your cleanse won't work.

If you aren't able to eliminate all of your regular meals, try to get rid of at least two. Replace your breakfast and lunch with a healthy smoothie made with either high amounts of protein, vegetables or greens. Then continue to eat dinner as you normally would. Try to keep your dinner a little smaller than you might normally eat. Remember you're trying to reduce your overall calories but you're also not trying to starve yourself. You can do this by cutting down portion sizes slightly or even using a smaller plate for your food that can trick your body into feeling full faster.

Your dinner should include protein and plenty of greens and vegetables. Try to avoid a lot of carbohydrates, junk food or sweet snacks here as well as you could find yourself experiencing side effects from mixing a lot of unhealthy foods with your detoxification. You don't want to experience those unpleasant side effects, and you definitely don't want to replace all the fat, calories and carbs that you're getting rid of in the rest of your diet. You'll feel pretty upset if your diet doesn't work out after all.

With this program also you should be drinking plenty of water. One gallon per day should be sufficient but if you feel yourself getting dehydrated feel free to drink more. If you get hungry while on this diet, you'll also want to consider drinking more water. When you drink a glass of water make sure that you wait for a short while, at least half an hour, before you eat something. Waiting helps the water to settle down into your stomach which will help you feel full faster when you start eating your meals (or your smoothies).

Another great thing about this is that you will be able to tell if you are actually hungry or if your body is just dehydrated. If it's not time for a meal and you start feeling hungry again try drinking one to two glasses of water or tea. Once you've finished them wait half an hour and see if you are still hungry. Quite frequently you'll find that you're no longer hungry because your body was just a little thirsty and didn't need to eat anything. In this instance, you've saved yourself from extra calories just by being a little patient.

For the last four days of your diet, you want to make sure that you are following the smoothie recipes below. You'll be surprised at how great they taste and you're also going to love the benefits of all that protein. Stick with mostly protein and vegetable shakes for your meals with a few fruit ones thrown in for sweetness. There are enough recipes here that you can actually have a new one for each meal even if you are able to eat only smoothies three days for the entire week. It's going to help you get enough healthy benefits as well and you're going to have all the variety that you really want in a diet.

Chapter 15

Equipment and Variation

Green Smoothies Storage What Equipment You'll Need

Powerful Blender and Green Smoothies

Obviously, a good blender is essential for making smoothies.

For successful creamy smoothies, a powerful blender is best.Otherwise, you may burn out the motor. But what if you only have an ordinary blender and want to avoid this? To work around the problem, you'll cut your vegetables into small pieces before putting them in the blender. Use a very sharp knife and finely chop everything you can, for example, celery stalks, and pieces of broccoli or apple wedges.

Obviously, if you have a food processor, go ahead and simply chop your vegetables before putting them in the blender. Several recipes for green smoothies recommend adding ice cubes or pieces of frozen fruit to make smoothies creamier. If your blender is not very powerful, bypass this step.

1. Use fresh fruit.
2. Thaw your fruits in advance if they are frozen.

3. Grind your ice at the beginning, alone, in a little water.
4. Soak walnuts, almonds or seeds a few hours before using.

It needs a lot of power to break up the cells of greens and unleash all of their nutrient power.So, you might want to get the Vitamix or Blend Tec. There are very similar and will do the job properly.

If you're Tight on Budget

Try NutriBullet. They say it is not as powerful as Vitamix or Blend Tec, and it will not last as long as they do, but still NutriBullet can make good green smoothies. Also, it's pretty cheap!

It doesn't have to have every bell and whistle, but get the best quality that you can afford.

Here are some things that you should consider:

- **How powerful the motor is** – You want a bit more of a powerful motor here because you will be chopping nuts and ice. Look for motors that are 500 watts and up.

- **How easy it is to wash** – Ideally, you should be able to disassemble the blade attachment and the actual jug of the blender from one another to be able to properly clean it out.

Simplicity in cleaning is pretty important – if the blender is tough to clean, it could end up being more trouble than it is worth to use it.If it takes too long to clean you, won't want to make your smoothies.

- **The strength of the jar** – I have used blenders with plastic jars and those with glass jars. In my experience, the glass one stands up better over time.

- **How many speeds it has** – With blending, you need only three settings – Pulse, and two different blending speed buttons.

My blender has these settings – I usually only use the lowest speed. Occasionally, when a piece of fruit or vegetable is stubborn, I use the pulse setting.
There are blenders out there that have several speed settings – this makes no difference, even my old, clapped out blender can blend a smoothie in less than a minute.

Variation

To give more flavor to your smoothies try new combinations. The possibilities are virtually endless. Here I will share with you the list of ingredients that I always keep on hand to vary the preparation of my green smoothies depending on my mood.

I look for frozen fruits that are natural without added sugar and frozen vegetables that are natural, without sauce or seasoning. Whenever possible, I buy organic products, otherwise I use a soaking solution to remove pesticides that are on the surface.

I do not use cow's milk, having been weaned off of it a long time ago. I also avoid soy milk. Consuming GMO soy does not really inspire me.

Ingredients followed by a letter tell you if they:

1. Stimulate metabolism **(M)**
2. Are Antioxidants **(A)**
3. Fight water retention **(R)**
4. Facilitate weight loss **(W)**
5. Contain good fats **(F)**.

Ingredients for green smoothies

1. Chopped garlic, fresh or preserved in oil **(A)**
2. Dill, fresh or dried
3. Bananas, fresh or frozen, cut into slices
4. Sticks of fresh celery **(R) (W)**
5. Almond Butter **(F)**
6. Macadamia nut butter **(F)**
7. Blueberries, fresh or frozen **(A)**
8. Frozen Broccoli **(A)**
9. Cinnamon **(M)**
10. Celery cubes, frozen **(R)**
11. Cucumber **(R) (W)**
12. Frozen mango cubes
13. Turmeric **(M) (A)**
14. Coconut Water
15. Spinach, fresh or frozen **(A)**
16. Fennel, fresh or dried. **(R)**
17. Strawberries, fresh or frozen
18. Raspberries, fresh or frozen
19. Unsalted sunflower seeds **(F)**
20. Dried Herbs de Provence
21. Olive oil **(F)**
22. Coconut oil **(F)**
23. Kale, fresh or frozen **(A) (R)**
24. Almond milk

25. Coconut Milk
26. Rice milk
27. Mint, fresh or dried
28. Unsalted cashews
29. Fresh parsley **(R) (W)**
30. Mixed berries, frozen
31. Cayenne Pepper **(M)**
32. Black pepper **(M)**
33. Garlic powder
34. Onion Powder
35. Tabasco **(M)**

Please note, if you put turmeric in your smoothie, do not forget to add black pepper and a tablespoon of coconut oil to boost the antioxidant properties of turmeric.

Chapter 16

Do Smoothies Really Work?

There has been a lot of press in the last few years about the benefits of drinking your nutrients in the form of smoothies and juices. There are those that say that juicing is lot better and that it will help you to lose weight. There are those who say that you have to eat "real" food and cannot "drink" your meals.Others say that smoothies are too high in calories.

The truth lies in the middle ground – with smoothies, you are drinking your food but you are still getting all the fiber that you would have in the "real" food.Most people actually start getting the right amounts of fiber for the first time in their lives because smoothies can be loaded with healthy foods and still taste good.

Smoothies do tend to have a lot of calories in them, but this is only if you make them incorrectly.If, on the other hand, you follow the recipes in this book and you make them with the right ingredients, you will find that they are low-calorie recipes!

Remember that your body does need lots of calories a day to sustain it – the big problem with fad diets is that they reduce the caloric intake to such an extent that your body feels as though it is starving and holds onto any calories that it can.

That is one of the reasons why you often gain weight so soon after going off one of the fad diets.

Super Smoothie to the Rescue

You want long-term weight loss, and overall health; Green Smoothies will help you achieve this goal. One way to curb hunger when dieting is adding fiber. You will get that much-needed fiber if you are making your smoothies correctly. You add a whole fruit or veggie into a smoothie – and this will maintain its already high fiber content!

The blending does break down some of the fiber content but, on the whole, you are still getting your daily dose of fiber. The impact on blood sugar levels is not nearly as great as in the case of, say, store-bought fruit juice.

You will get enough of each type of fiber – soluble and insoluble.

Soluble fiber is absorbed into the blood stream and helps to mop up excess LDL cholesterol, keeping your heart healthier. Oats are a great source of soluble fiber, and that is why you will see them in some of the recipes.

Insoluble fiber is just as important – it makes you feel fuller for longer and it is essential for the health of the good bacteria in our guts; it helps the food move as it should through the digestive tract and helps you stay regular.

Vegetables and fruits contain some insoluble fiber and some soluble fiber.Let's face it - nature wants us to eat fruit and veggies whole.

Smoothies offer a bit of a compromise – you get adequate fiber and a shot of vitamins and minerals in quantities that are closer to what nature originally intended, in a convenient liquid form. Your average smoothie contains about the same amount of food that you should be eating in terms of a healthy, natural diet. The high levels of nutrients in the smoothies give your body what it needs to repair itself, and so you will find that cravings go away. The fresh ingredients in the smoothies are packed with antioxidants and so will help to fight the signs of aging and inflammation. They will also help to flush toxins out of your system. Additionally, you won't feel as hungry as you used to because smoothies are very filling.

You can even tailor the types of smoothies that you drink so that you get the optimal benefits for your own personal condition – do you have a lot of problems with inflammation? Make sure you add plenty of nuts and seeds. Need to get rid of gout? Celery is great at balancing the levels of uric acid in your system.

Smoothies taste good, are easy to prepare and fit in perfectly if you need to eat on the run.

They are the perfect way to lose weight – you just need to put the right ingredients in.

Chapter 17

How to Make a Perfect Green Smoothie

You can make a green smoothie using almost any of the fruits and vegetables you have in your refrigerator – you can also use add-ins like honey, nuts or seeds and fruit juice to improve the flavor. Below you will find a general green smoothie recipe with a step-by-step guide to begin making smoothies at home.

Step 1: Choose a Base

The base of your green smoothie is what gives it texture – frozen bananas or fresh avocado are great options. Other frozen fruits work as well, but the resulting texture may not be as smooth

Step 2: Choose Your Greens

Consider leafy greens, fresh herbs, and other green vegetables. Remember that whatever ingredient you use the most of in your green smoothie is likely to be the flavor you taste the most as well

Step 3: Choose Additional Flavors

If you don't like the idea of a spinach-flavored smoothie, throw in some frozen berries or a sliced apple to improve the flavor. Don't forget that nut butter and raw nuts can also be used to flavor smoothies

Step 4: Add Liquid

- not all green smoothies will require liquid but adding some liquid will help to give you that smooth, blended texture
- consider organic fruit juices, nonfat yogurt, non-dairy milk or plain water

Step 5: Add Sweetener (optional)

To further mask the flavor of whatever vegetables you use in your green smoothie, you can also choose to add a tablespoon of sweeteners like honey, maple syrup or agave nectar

Step 6: Blend and Garnish

After choosing all of your ingredients all that is left for you to do is combine them in the blender and blend smooth.To dress up your green smoothie, garnish it with a fresh berry or a sprinkle of seeds

Chapter 18

Long-Term Solution of Green Smoothies

The beauty of this plan is that you only need to stick to it for nine days. It is not recommended that you continue for longer than this.

You will now no doubt be fired up and looking for ways to keep the "buzz" going.

The good news is that you have now broken some of your bad eating habits and have seen the astonishing benefits that come from eating in this manner.

For optimal benefits, it is a good idea to slowly start transitioning back to a more "normal" diet.

Here are some ideas to help you along that journey:

- Your system has had no solid foods over the last nine days so you want to ease back into things slowly. Start by introducing one light meal a day in place of one of the smoothies.

- This meal should consider mostly of raw vegetables and should be a light meal. You also need to add in some protein. Smoked chicken, steamed fish, salmon or boiled eggs are a good way to keep the meal light and healthy.

- Keep the food simple – add flavor with spices rather than with creamy and rich sauces.

- After a week or so, you can start swopping out your second smoothie for a meal – again, keep to simple foods.

- After a week like this, you can swop out the last smoothie if you want to. Many people opt to leave at least one meal as a smoothie a day – it helps with energy and is convenient.

A Healthy Diet

If you go back to eating as you were before, you will simply start to feel sick and will start to gain weight again. It makes no sense to fall back into bad habits. Fortunately, your body now has a taste for the healthy food, and it will want more of the same.

Make sure that you have a diet rich in raw fruit and vegetables and eat protein at every meal to further your weight loss goals.

Try to follow a whole food approach when looking at what foods to buy - was the food made by nature or made by a factory? Highly processed foods have few, if any nutrients and should be avoided as much as possible.

You should also have learned that healthy food does not need to be bland and boring. Use the herbs and spices that you have learned about here in cooking. Look into making herbal teas to continue the detox process more gently – Fennel, for example, is an excellent diuretic.

- Parsley tea is a blood cleanser and bone builder.
- Cumin tea will help ease digestive upsets.
- Alfalfa tea is alkalizing.

The list goes on and on - do yourself a favor and look into herbal teas and what they can do for you.

Just remember, you should not take herbal tea for longer than ten days in a row. Take a break for about a week and start up again if you want to.

At the very least, you need to maintain your 3 cups of green tea a day. Try livening it up a bit with mint or lemon or get adventurous and add a bit of cumin or nutmeg.

You should still be drinking your lemon juice in warm water every morning. Try kicking that up a few notches by adding a ¼ teaspoon cinnamon (to regulate blood sugar) and a ¼ teaspoon cayenne pepper (to rev up your metabolism).

I'm not going to lie – it does not taste that great, but you do get used to the taste pretty quickly, so hang in there.

If you really and truly find that you cannot get used to the taste, have plain lemon water again and mix the cayenne pepper and cinnamon to a teaspoon of honey and take it like that. It helps it taste a little sweeter.

Probably the hardest part of any diet is staying healthy after it's over. This program is intended to be acleansing for you which means you won't continue with it forever. But that means you need to understand how to keep your weight under control, which can be extremely difficult for a number of different people. You need to make sure that you understand the basics of being healthy and definitely that you understand some of the important aspects of eating right, exercise and much more. That's the only way you'll keep the weight off.

Once you finish your detox and cleanse you're going to be at your best. This is when you'll be able to lose the most weight because your body isn't trying to make up for all the toxins and it's not struggling to function under the weight of all those toxins either. Once you've cleansed them out you won't have to worry about them as much and you'll be able to lose a lot of weight much more quickly than you would at any other point in time. This is because you are only getting the nutrients that your body needs and your body isn't hogging them all as much as it would under other circumstances. The first thing you need to make sure that you do is eat right. You want to continue drinking a gallon or more of water or tea each day. You can add some natural fruit juices, but try to limit the amount of these as well. Adding juices increases the amount of sugar in drinks, and that is going to increase the number of calories that you consume. Added calories will increase the amount of weight that you put on. You need to keep your weight down after all so you can continue to be healthy.

When you eat your meals, you need to make sure that you are getting enough protein, enough fruits, and enough vegetables as well. To be truly healthy you're going to want to decrease the amount of protein compared to everything else. Increasing the amount of fruit and vegetables gets you a lot more vitamins and minerals that you get from your food. As a result of this you're going to improve your overall health, and you're going to make sure that you don't put on a lot of weight either.

What's really important to consider is what type of fruit and vegetables you're including as well. Vegetables are going to help you in any way you use them. You can cook these foods however you choose though remember that raw or blanched vegetables are going to be the best for you. If you bake you will still be better off than if you fry any of your foods, whether it's vegetables or the protein you have. If you eat fruit, on the other, hand you need to make sure that you are eating them raw without adding a lot of extra things like sugar or syrup.

Fruit is healthy for you in its raw state without a lot of additives because it's going to allow you to get vitamins and minerals. You should avoid adding a lot of sugar or sweets to your fruit; you will diminish their healthy benefits. Of that, the benefits that you do get, they are mitigated a lot by the additives. These are going to counteract your potential benefits because you're getting unhealthy things that make you gain more weight instead of losing it like you're hoping to. They also increase the toxins that you get in your body.

You may need to look into the amount of calories that you really need for your body during your day. You want to make sure that you are getting enough but that you're not eating too much. For women, the generally accepted calorie intake is around 1800 +; while for men the general calorie intake is 2000 +. Remember that this is to maintain your current weight (and it will depend on what your current weight is as well as your current exercise level).

If you're planning to lose some weight, you should talk to your doctor about what is a safe amount of calories for your situation. They will be able to help you figure out your calorie intake as well as the specific vitamins and minerals that you need to stay healthy and the type of exercise that you should be doing. You won't be able to lose weight and stay in great shape if you aren't adding at least a little exercise into your regular plan. Adding in exercise is going to be important because it helps you burn some calories. It also helps to keep your body in better shape. If you're exercising at least 30 minutes at least every other day you should be able to get some benefits from the process and you'll be able to ensure that your calorie intake isn't too much. If you want to get into better shape you can increase the amount of time you spend exercising or the amount of days that you exercise. Just make sure that you're pushing yourself and getting as much as you can from your exercise.

The key is going to be continuing to detox frequently. You want to make sure that you detox your body through this method or a very similar one at least 4 times per year. This means you're going to go through a full week of detox every quarter, or every 3 months. This is going to allow you to reduce the amount of toxins that are getting into your body through normal life. Keep this detox on hand so that you can revert back to it when it's time for your next detox. If you start feeling slowed down or drawn down you can start a new Detox then as well.

30 green smoothie

1# Coco papaya twister thick green smoothies

Yield: 4 glasses
Ingredients
1. 2 cups ice cubes
2. 2 cups coconut water
3. 6 tablespoon dried pitted dates
4. 2 cups ripe papaya chunks
5. 1 cup chopped kale leaves

Preparation:
- Blend ice cubes, coconut water and kale leaves until smooth.
- Add remaining ingredients, and blend until smooth. Enjoy!

To improve taste – you can put almonds 4 table spoon almonds. Soak them first and remove the skin of almond to make them more digestible

Garnish:

Top of each glass place slice of dried pitted date, and papaya chunk.

Smoothie secretes

This smoothie has kale it is low in calorie, high in fiber and has zero fat. Kale is rich source of iron, Vitamin, and kale is powerful antioxidants it will also help you with cardiovascular support and Vitamin A not only you are drinking a tasty smoothie but in fact this will help you to detoxify your body.

Nutritional information-

1. Calories = 237
2. Carbohydrate= 54 g
3. Protein = 5g
4. Fiber = 11g

2# avocado buster limes –

Yield -1 glass
Ingredients
1. 6 piece ice cubes
2. 1 cup Unsweetened coconut water
3. ½ avocado fruit
4. 2 whole limes
5. 1 sliced apple.
6. 1tablespoon honey.

Preparation:
- Pluck out the leaves of the spinach. Discard stems.
- Remove seed of avocado. Using a spoon, scoop out flesh.
- Peal and quarter limes.
- Cut apple into half –inch slices.
- Blend ice, coconut water and avocado until smooth.
- Add remaining ingredients, and blend until smooth. Enjoy!
- Pour into glass and drink fresh.

Garnish:

Top of each glass place thin apple slice.

Smoothie secret:

Avocado is a green part of this smoothie It will help you with antioxidant carotenoids, vitamin e and vitamin c it is also helpful for skin care also and this smoothies help you with diabetes and arthritis. More of a juice than a smoothie (because of the ingredient's low fiber content), this invigorating frappe alkalizes and hydrates the body. That is why this drink is perfect for right after a strenuous workout or when it's hot outside. In fact, I highly recommend you add this to the menu for all of your midsummer picnics and sporting events. It's tasty, light, and refreshing.

Nutritional information-

1. Calories = 218
2. Carbohydrate= 44 g
3. Protein = 7g
4. Fiber = 21g

3# Broccoli apple combo smoothie

Yield: 2 glasses

Ingredients
- ½ cup broccoli heads
- 1 cup spinach
- 1 green apple.
- 1 orange.
- 1 cup Coconut milk
- ½ cup chopped cantaloupe
- 1 cup ice cubes

Preparation-
1. Wash the spinach under running water.
2. Peel orange. Separate into segments.
3. Peel and core apple. Cut them into ½ inch cubes.
4. Put all ingredients into blender and blend it for 4 minutes at high speed until it all mix up well.
5. Pour into glass and serve it.

Smoothie secret:

Cantaloupe is the most popular variety of melon in the United States and it's easy to see why. Succulently sweet and a great source of beta-carotene, a powerful antioxidant, this fruit is nothing less than a big ball of joy. Here I've dressed it up with a handful of herbs and a touch of extra sweetness. Fresh spinach leaves are rich source of several vital anti-oxidant vitamins like vitamin A, vitamin C, and flavonoid poly phenolic antioxidants such as lutein, zea-xanthin and beta also spinach will help you with your weight reduction.

Nutritional information-

1. Calories = 240
2. Carbohydrate= 67g
3. Protein = 10g
4. Fiber = 12g

4# Cool kale mint smoothie

Yield -2 glass
Ingredients

1. Cup chopped kale leaves
2. 15 pieces mint leaves
3. 4 whole pitted dates
4. 2 tablespoon raw cashew
5. 1 ½ cup coconut milk.

Preparation

- Put all ingredients in a blender. Whiz on high speed until smooth.
- Pour into glasses and serve immediately.

Make it better-
If you like to change the taste try to put 1 cup ice cube for cold treat.

Smoothie secret:

Kale is such a delicate and beautiful little green. Kale is a very versatile and nutritious green leafy vegetable. It is a widely popular vegetable since ancient Greek and Roman times for its low fat, no cholesterol but health benefiting anti-oxidant properties. It adds a peppery flavor to this smooth drink that is very reminiscent of horseradish. I love everything about this smoothie and with the little kale leaves for garnish, it's as gorgeous as it is tasty.

Nutritional information-

1. Calories = 286
2. Carbohydrate= 74 g
3. Protein = 9g
4. Fiber = 9g

5# Honey avocado thunder smoothie

Yield: 1 glass
Ingredients
1. 1cup chopped zucchini.
2. ½ cup sliced cucumber
3. ½ avocado fruit
4. 3 whole limes
5. 2 tablespoon Natural honey
6. 6 pieces ice cubes

Preparation:
- Washed vegetables and fruits thoroughly.
- Cut cucumber into half-inch slices.
- Remove seed of avocado. Using a spoon, scoop out flesh from the peeling.
- Peel and quarter limes.
- In a blender, place cucumber, avocado, chopped zucchini and lime. Add ice cubes and 2 table spoon honey.
- Blend all ingredients until smooth.
- Pour into a glass and drink fresh.

Smoothie secret:

Adding fruits and vegetables that alkalize the body help you to stay balanced and nip illnesses in the bud. This smoothie includes some of the most powerful alkalizing vegetables like cucumber and avocado, which is exactly how this drink got its alkalizing super hero identity. Zucchini is a very good source of potassium, an important intra-cellular electrolyte. Potassium is a heart-friendly electrolyte and helps bring the reduction in blood pressure and heart rates by countering pressure-effects of sodium.

Nutritional information-

1. Calories = 227
2. Carbohydrate= 4 8g
3. Protein = 12g
4. Fiber = 15g

6# 3Amigo green smoothie

Yield: 1 glass
Ingredients:
1. 1 cup romaine lettuce
2. 1 medium sized apple
3. 1 medium sized avocado
4. ¼ lemon fruit
5. 1 tablespoon slice ginger
6. A pinch of salt
7. ½ cup distilled water

Preparation:
- Rinse romaine lettuce in running water.
- Without peeling, core and segment apples.
- Peel ginger and cut into thin slices.
- Peel lemon and removes seeds.
- Cut avocado into halves, remove seed and scoop out flesh using a tablespoon.
- Put all ingredients in a blender.
- Whiz on high speed until well mixed and smooth.
- Pour into a glass and enjoy.

Smoothie secret:

When you think ginger, you may think of salsa, but this smoothie is anything but. This zesty herb adds a tantalizing freshness that tickles your taste buds while purifying your body. Ginger has been used to cleanse the blood of heavy metals like mercury and lead. You can feel great unwinding with this smoothie because it fills you up with healthy fats and fiber while taking a bit of toxic weight off of your shoulders. Lettuce is a rich source of vitamin K. Vitamin K has a potential role in the bone metabolism where it thought to increase bone mass by promoting osteotrophic activity inside the bone cells. It also has established role in Alzheimer's disease patients by limiting neuronal damage in the brain.

Nutritional information-

1. Calories = 297
2. Carbohydrate= 84 g
3. Protein = 7g
4. Fiber = 19g

7# Tangy minty green smoothie

Yield: 1 glass
Ingredient

1. 10 leaves coriander
2. 10 leaves of mint
3. 10 leaves of sweet basil
4. 2 Ripe orange
5. ½ small avocado fruit
6. ½ cup cucumber slices
7. Juice of ½ lime fruit
8. ½ cup distilled water

Preparation:

- Peel orange and separate them, remove seeds.
- Scoop the flesh from the avocado fruit.
- Slice cucumber in to half-inch thickness.
- Put all ingredients in a blender in this order mint, basil, coriander, orange, avocado, cucumber, lime juice. Blend on high speed until smooth.
- Pour into glass and serve fresh.

Smoothie secret:

Our modern day lives expose us to a myriad of toxins. Whether it is car exhaust or pesticides, it all adds to our toxic load. Beets are thought to have the amazing ability to cleanse poisons like these from the body. This simple frappe will refresh you, while alkalizing and purifying your body of the toxins we accumulate on a daily basis. Green part of this smoothie is avocado which will help you with your weight loss and skin benefit.

Nutritional information-

1. Calories = 259
2. Carbohydrate= 37 g
3. Protein = 6g
4. Fiber = 13g

8# Apple broccoli smoothie

Yield: 2 galas
Ingredient
1. 1 cup Swiss chard.
2. ½ cup broccoli heads
3. 1 cup ice cubes
4. 1 big sized apple
5. 1 cup watermelon.

Preparation:
- Rinse broccoli heads & Swiss card under running water.
- Peel and core apple. Cut into ½ inch cubes.
- Remove seeds and cut watermelon into one inch cubes.
- Put all ingredients in a blender. Blend on high speed until thoroughly combined.
- Pour into a glass and serve.

Smoothie secret:

This frappe is meant to be shared. Watermelons, due to their large size and short shelf life, are not a fruit you can eat all by yourself. For this reason, I highly recommend making this smoothie for a party or get together. You can use the entire watermelon in one shot while delighting guests with a healthy and energizing treat. This smoothie also contains anti oxidant and vitamin A which is very good for your eye.

Nutritional information-

1. Calories = 232
2. Carbohydrate= 64 g
3. Protein = 8g
4. Fiber = 9g

9# zucchini pineapple thick smoothie

Yield: 1 glass

Ingredients:
1. 1 cup zucchini
2. 1 cup pineapple
3. ½ tablespoon chopped ginger
4. 2 whole pitted dates
5. ½ distilled water
6. 1 cup ice cubes

Preparation:
1. In a blender, add zucchini and water. Blend until smooth.
2. Add all remaining ingredients and process until blended smoothly.
3. Pour into a glass and enjoy.

Smoothie secret:

Growing up, my mom always treated us to a loaf of moist zucchini bread in midsummer when her garden was bursting with summer squash. This smoothie is a take on this bread, showing zucchini's sweeter side. It's rich and delicious; you'd never be able to guess that there is a healthy vegetable in the mix. This smoothie also contains moderate levels of B-complex group of vitamins like thiamin, pyridoxine, riboflavin and minerals like iron, manganese, phosphorus, and zinc. Zucchini also help us with these compounds help scavenge harmful oxygen-derived free radicals and reactive oxygen species (ROS) from the body that play a role in aging and various disease processes.

Nutritional information-

1. Calories = 245
2. Carbohydrate= 51 g
3. Protein = 2g
4. Fiber = 21g

10# BB magic smoothie

Yield: 1 glass

Ingredients:
1. 1 cup broccoli
2. 2 cups diced ripe bananas
3. ½ cup distilled water
4. ½ cup ice cubes

Preparation:
- Rinse broccoli in running water and clean thoroughly.
- Peel bananas and cut into 1-inch slices.
- Put all ingredients in a blender and whiz until smooth.
- Pour into a glass and enjoy.

Smoothie secret:
Your mom always told you to eat your broccoli and this smoothie will definitely do the trick. It's just like the famous juice, but with the added benefit of fiber. And with so many vitamins and minerals, it's like a multivitamin in a glass. Smart and delicious, with every sip of this smoothie, you make your mother proud!

Nutritional information-

1. Calories = 230
2. Carbohydrate= 62g
3. Protein = 6g
4. Fiber = 18g

11# all fruit power smoothie

Yield: 1 glass

Ingredients:

1. 2 pieces apples
2. 1 piece banana
3. 1 cup dices pineapple
4. ½ piece cucumber
5. 1 cup water.

Preparation:

- Peel, core and cut apples into 1-inch cubes.
- Peel banana and cut into 1-inch slices.
- Without peeling, cut cucumbers into 1-inch cubes.
- Place all ingredients in a blender and whiz until smooth.
- Pour into a glass and serve immediately.

Smoothie secret:

My favorite desserts are often an inspiration for new smoothie endeavors, and this one is no different. The all-too-familiar flavor combination of apple, pineapple, and cucumber make me think of pineapple cake. With no gluten or refined sugars, I think this is even better. Try the variation below and you will believe too.

Nutritional information-

1. Calories = 269
2. Carbohydrate= 36 g
3. Protein = 11g
4. Fiber = 18g

12# cocaberry super detox smoothie.

Yield: 2 glasses

Ingredients:
1. 2 cups romaine lettuce.
2. 1 ½ cups fresh blackberry.
3. 3 piece pitted date (pre- soaked)
4. ½ cup almond milk.
5. ½ cup coconut milk.
6. ½ cup ice cubes

Preparation:
- Blend romaine lettuce, milk and water until smooth.
- Add in the rest of ingredients and continue blending until thoroughly mixed.
- Pour into tall glasses and serve immediately.

Smoothie secret:
Can you say super fruit? Blackberries are a powerhouse of health-boosting nutrients like phytochemicals and antioxidants, which may help fight cancer. But that's not even why I recommend this smoothie for weight loss. This is the smoothie to grab when you are craving something sweet, but don't want to go overboard. It helps you get your sugar fix without cheating.

Nutritional information-

1. Calories = 220
2. Carbohydrate= 64 g
3. Protein = 8g
4. Fiber = 32g

13# honey brewed green smoothie

Yield: 1 glass

Ingredients:
1. ½ cup spinach
2. ½ cup sliced apple
3. 1 tablespoon raw honey
4. ½ cup freshly brewed green tea
5. ½ cup low- fat yogurt
6. 1 cup ice cubes

Preparation:
- Peel apple and sliced it.
- Cool brewed green tea to room temperature.
- In blender, add spinach, yogurt and green tea. Blend until smooth.
- Add all remaining ingredients and process until smooth.
- Pour into glasses and serve immediately.

Smoothie secret:
If you've never had the pleasure of sinking your teeth into a jicama before, you are in for a pleasant surprise. This root vegetable is crisp with a refreshing, while at the same time slightly starchy flavor. It here with a plethora of fresh citrus flavors. This smoothie is bright and delicious with a ton of beneficial fiber.

Nutritional information-

1. Calories = 245
2. Carbohydrate= 51 g
3. Protein = 2g
4. Fiber = 21g

14# kale oats power smoothie

Yield: 2 glasses

Ingredient:

1. ½ Cup parsley leaves
2. ½ cup oats
3. ½ kale leaves
4. A pinch of salt
5. ½ cup unsweetened coconut milk
6. 1 cup water
7. ½ cup ice cubes

Preparation:

- Blend kale and parsley leaves with water.
- When smooth, add oats, salt, coconut milk and ice cubes and blend until fully mixed.
- Pour into a glass and serve.

Smoothie secret:

Kale levees are often dubbed a super food and it's easy to see why. Each little nugget offers a sizable dose of magnesium as well as fiber and healthy fats. Chemicals in parsley leaves also have been thought to give you a euphoric feeling. Your kids will have no problem falling in love with this mouth-watering smoothie. It has kale which is rich in Zea-xanthin, an important dietary carotenoid, is selectively absorbed into the retinal macula lutea in the eyes where it is thought to provide antioxidant and protective light-filtering functions. Thus, it helps prevent retinal detachment and offer protection against "age-related macular degeneration related macular degeneration disease" (ARMD) in the elderly.

Nutritional information-

1. Calories = 264
2. Carbohydrate= 73 g
3. Protein = 22g
4. Fiber = 21g

15# piena milk berry smoothie

Yield: 2 glasses
Ingredients:
1. ½ cup broccoli
2. ½ cup blueberries
3. ½ cup pineapple
4. ½ cup oats
5. 1 tablespoon sunflower seeds
6. One cup non- dairy milk of your choice
7. 4 strawberry
8. ½ cup water
9. ½ ice cubes

Preparation:
- Put ice cubes, water, broccoli and oats in a blender. Blend until smooth.
- Add milk, blueberries, bananas and sunflower seeds. Blend until smooth
- Pour into a glass immediately.

Smoothie secret:

To our ancient hunter-gatherer ancestors, berries were the ultimate treat. From branch to belly, these little bundles of joy provided a powerful dose of energy along with antioxidants and their fair share of fiber. Today you can reap the same benefits! This smoothie is homage to our favorite snack with a combination of tasty berries freshened up with some delicious herbs. As for as green part it has broccoli and that is a storehouse of many phyto-nutrients such as *thiocyanates, indoles, sulforaphane, isothiocyanates* and *flavonoids like beta-carotene cryptoxanthin, lutein, and zea-xanthin.* Studies have shown that these compounds by modifying positive signaling at molecular receptor levels help protect from prostate, colon, urinary bladder, pancreatic, and breast cancers.

Nutritional information-

1. Calories = 242
2. Carbohydrate=34 g
3. Protein =17
4. Fiber = 9g

16# Brussels honey lemon tangy smoothie

Yield: 2 glasses
Ingredients:
1. 1 cup cucumber
2. 1 orange
3. 2 tablespoon Chia seeds
4. ½ cup lemon juice
5. 2 tablespoon honey
6. ½ Brussels sprouts
7. ½ cup ice cubes

Preparation:
- Cut cucumber without peeling in to 1-inch slice.
- Peel orange remove them into segments.
- Put all ingredients into the blender and blend until smooth.
- Pour into glass and drink fresh.

Smoothie secret:

This smoothie is inspired by a mouthwatering salad that you would find at a high-end restaurant. It's is so deliciously sweet, though, that you'd never guess there is a leafy green in the mix. It's a great fix for those times when you are cravings something sweet. With the fiber, iron, and vitamin C that this drink offers, you will never have to feel guilty about giving in. Brussels sprouts contain glucoside, sinigrin. Early laboratory studies suggest that *sinigrin* help protect from colon cancers by destroying pre-cancerous cells.Brussel sprouts are an excellent source of vitamin C; 100 g sprouts provide about 85 mg or 142% of RDA. Together with other antioxidant vitamins such as vitamin A and E, it helps protect the body by trapping harmful free radicals.

Nutritional information-

1. Calories = 232
2. Carbohydrate=39 g
3. Protein =13
4. Fiber = 20g

17# water melon cantaloupe fun smoothie

Yield: 2 glasses

Ingredients:
1. ½ Cup Cantaloupe
2. 1 cup water melon
3. 1 celery medium sized
4. 5 mint leaves
5. 1 cup diced banana
6. ½ cucumber
7. 1 cup ice cubes

Preparation:
- Peel and cut cantaloupe in to 1-inch cube.
- Remove seed from water melon.
- Put all ingredient in blender and blend them until smooth
- Pour into glass garnish it with mint levees, drink it fresh.

Smoothie secret:

While we eat water melon all the time in this country, they are actually native to China. Wherever they come from, they are sweet, juicy, and packed with potassium. The water melon in these smoothies have been spiced up with a sprinkling of exotic spices mint leaves. There's no better way to enjoy this decadent fruit. This smoothie reduces inflammation. If you are suffering from joint pains, lung infections, asthma, or acne, eating more celery will bring much-needed relief. It helps you calm down: and work as stress-relief? Oh yes! The minerals in this smoothie, especially magnesium and essential oill in it, soothe the nervous system.

Nutritional information-

1. Calories = 238
2. Carbohydrate=53 g
3. Protein =9
4. Fiber = 15g

18 # green spinach peaches twist smoothie

Yield: 2

Ingredients:
1. ½ cup spinach
2. ½ cup Brussels sprouts.
3. 2 medium peaches
4. 2 medium banana
5. ½ cup green tea.

6. 1 cup Fresh raspberries

Preparation:
- Rinse spinach & Brussels sprouts in running water and clean thoroughly.
- Remove seed from peaches with the tablespoon.
- First put green in the blender with green tea whiz until smooth
- Now time to put rest of the ingredient into blender and blend until smooth.
- Pour it in the glass and drink fresh.

Smoothie secret:

This frappe is one of my all-time favorite drinks. If you are a green tea lover, you will go nuts for it. The grassy flavor of the spinach accentuates the tea perfectly and grapes add a subtle sweetness. The antioxidants, vitamins, and minerals in this tasty concoction are just icing on the cake. Spinach is store house for many phyto-nutrients that have health promotional and disease prevention properties.

Nutritional information-

1. Calories = 252
2. Carbohydrate=46 g
3. Protein =3g
4. Fiber = 20g

19# green thunder in my smoothie cup

Yield: 2 glasses

Ingredients
1. 1 cup chopped avocado.
2. 1 cup watercress
3. Medium sized cucumber
4. ½ cup lime juice
5. 1 cup ice cubes
6. Pinch of Sea salt

Preparation:
- Scoop the flesh from the avocado fruit.
- Without peeling cucumber cut it in to 1-inch pieces.
- Put all ingredients in the blender. Start on low, and then increase the speed to high. Blend until smooth.
- Pour into glass and taste it sour and salty taste.

Smoothie secret:
I am a huge fan of Indian cuisine. With the combination of warm spices and decadent fruits, chutneys are definitely included in my Indian favorites. That is exactly what inspired me to make this smoothie. Sea salt is an Indian favorite

and it pairs perfectly with the succulently sweet flavor that cucumber has to offer. The best part is that watercress it is also rich source of minerals like copper, calcium, potassium, magnesium, manganese and phosphorus. Potassium is an important component of cell and body fluids that helps controlling heart rate and blood pressure by countering effects of sodium. Manganese is used by the body as a co-factor for the antioxidant enzyme, SUPEROXIDE DISMUTASE. Calcium is required as bone/teeth mineral and in the regulation of heart and skeletal muscle activity.

Nutritional information-

1. Calories = 272
2. Carbohydrate=42 g
3. Protein =6g
4. Fiber =19g

20# Simple but strong berries lettuce smoothie

Yield-2 glass

Ingredients:
1. 1 cup chopped romaine lettuce
2. 2 cups fresh blackberries
3. ½ tablespoon lemon zest
4. 1 large banana
5. 5 mint leaves
6. 1 cup ice cubes
7. ½ cup chopped zucchini

Preparation:
- First put chopped romaine lettuce & and zucchini in blender and whiz until smooth.
- Now peel and cut in to slice banana.
- Put all ingredients in the blender, and blend them until smooth
- Pour it into a glass and drink fresh.

Smoothie secret:

Forget the cocktail! Renew yourself after a long day with this delicious smoothie. Relax knowing that you will be bolstering up your immune system with vitamin C and tons of antioxidants. Better yet, invite friends over and share this mock-tail with them. They'll be shocked and delighted when they learn that they just drank a boat load of healthy vegetables! Romaine lettuce Fresh leaves contain good amounts folates and vitamin C. Folates are part of co-factors in the enzyme metabolism required for DNA synthesis and therefore, play a vital role in prevention of the neural tube defects in the baby (fetus) during pregnancy.

Nutritional information-

1. Calories = 278
2. Carbohydrate=52 g
3. Protein =9g
4. Fiber =27g

21# Sweet coco spinach smoothie

Yield: 2 glasses

Ingredients
1. 1 whole lime
2. ½ cup young coconut meat
3. 1 cup baby spinach
4. 1 cup Swiss chard leaves
5. ½ peaches
6. ½ avocado
7. ½ medium sized cucumber
8. 1 cup coconut water

Preparation:
- Wash spinach, Swiss chard and cucumber thoroughly in running water. Chop the leaves and cut the cucumber without peeling into 1-inch cubes.
- Scoop out the flesh of the avocado discard the seed.
- Peel lime and quarter.
- In a blender, mix spinach Swiss chard and coconut water until smooth.
- Add remaining ingredients and blend until smooth and mixed thoroughly.

- Pour into a glass and enjoy fresh.

Smoothie secret:

Ever had a batch of guacamole that was so tasty you with you could just drink it up with a straw? Here's your chance. Even if you don't fall into that category, you will love this smoothie. It's light and refreshing, yet at the same time smooth and satisfying. All of your favorite guacamole ingredients are teamed up in just the right amounts to make for a delicious spicy treat. Swiss chard is an excellent source of antioxidant vitamin, vitamin-C. Its fresh leaves provide about 33% of recommended levels per 100 g. As a powerful water-soluble antioxidant, vitamin C helps to quench free radicals and reactive oxygen species (ROS) through its reduction potential properties. Research studies suggest that regular consumption of foods rich in vitamin C help maintain normal connective tissue, prevent iron deficiency, and also help the human body develop resistance against infectious agents by boosting immunity.

Nutritional information-

1. Calories = 239
2. Carbohydrate=36 g
3. Protein =12g
4. Fiber =7g

22# Rich mango- broccoli milk smoothie

Yield: 2 glasses

Ingredients:
1. 1 cup almond milk
2. ½ cup coconut milk
3. 1 whole medium sized ripe mango
4. ½ cup frozen banana
5. 4 medium sized broccoli heads
6. 1 cup ice cubes

Preparation:
- Wash and prepare all ingredients. Peel the mango, remove the seed and slice onto 2- inch cubes. Juice the lime fruit.
- Pour coconut milk into blender & almond milk add mango, banana and lime juice. Add broccoli last.
- Blend all ingredients on high speed until smoothie reaches a creamy consistency (This will take about 30 seconds to process).
- Pour into a glass and serve fresh.

Smoothie secret:

Ready to indulge? This smoothie feels like dessert while filling you and your family up for the long day ahead. And the best part, it tastes just like pie! This recipe is perfect for kids, too. They'd never guess that they are fueling up on fiber, beta-carotene, healthy fats, and antioxidants. It's a treat for your taste buds as well as your health. This smoothie is very low in calorie it is rich in dietary fiber, minerals, vitamins, and anti-oxidants that have proven health benefits.

Nutritional information-

1. Calories = 287
2. Carbohydrate=27g
3. Protein =16g
4. Fiber =5g

23# sweet pink kale smoothie

Yield: 2 Glasses
Ingredients:
1. 2 cups chopped kale leaves
2. 1 large whole orange
3. ½ cup pine apple
4. ½ cup slice bananas
5. 1/3 cup strawberries
6. ½ cup plain yogurt
7. 1 cup ice cubes

Preparation:
1. Peel oranges and divide into segments. Remove seeds if there any.
2. Put all ingredients in a blender. Puree until smooth.
3. Pour into glasses and serve immediately.

Smoothie secret:

Not a fan of kale leaves? Drink your this nutritious vegetable instead of eating it and still reap all the benefits. This smoothie is a chock-full of vitamin C, A, and K. The best part is that you can barely taste the kale! You'd be amazed at what you can sneak into a smoothie with a foundation of delicious, yet healthful, ingredients like yogurt, strawberries, and bananas. This smoothie will help you with B-complex group of vitamin b-6 , thiamin, pantothenic acid, etc., that are essential for substrate metabolism in the body.

Nutritional information-

1. Calories = 282
2. Carbohydrate=23g
3. Protein =13g
4. Fiber =7g

24# 3fruit one green thick smoothie

Yield: 2 glasses
Ingredient:
1. ½ cup Brussels sprouts.
2. ½ cup ripe mango chunks
3. ½ cup diced ripe bananas
4. ½ cup muesli
5. ½ cup pineapple
6. 1 tablespoon sesame seeds
7. ¼ cup pitted dates
8. ½ cup non-dairy milk
9. ½ cup ice cubes

Preparation:

- Place water, milk, muesli and l Brussels sprouts in a blender. Mix thoroughly.
- Add remaining ingredients and continue blending until smooth
- Pour into glass and drink fresh.

Smoothie secret:

Break out the beach chairs and sun hats; it's time for a trip to the beach! While you and your family may not have the opportunity to step out of your house today, but this smoothie will make you feel like you are in the Bahamas. It features a mouthwatering combination of luscious tropical fruits. They are packed with antioxidants, and the best part, they are absolutely delicious!

Nutritional information-

1. Calories = 276
2. Carbohydrate=17g
3. Protein =20g
4. Fiber =12g

25# dairy berry green smoothie

Yield: 1 glass
Ingredients:
1. ½ cup spinach
2. ½ cup sliced bananas
3. ½ cup blueberries
4. ½ cup non- dairy milk
5. ½ cup oats
6. 1 tablespoon sunflower seeds
7. ½ cup ice cubes
8. ½ cup water

Preparation:
- Put ice cubes, water, spinach and oats in a blender. Blend on high speed until mixed.
- Add milk blueberries, bananas and sunflower seeds. Blend until smooth.
- Pour into a tall glass and serve.

Smoothie secret:
Ready for something a little outside the box? This mouthwatering smoothie is a combination of tart blueberries, sweet banana, and an effervescent twist. Sunflower seeds just a little something that will leave you thinking and wanting more! Try sharing this daring drink and see if your friends and family can guess the secret ingredient.

Nutritional information-

1. Calories = 266
2. Carbohydrate=19g
3. Protein =24g
4. Fiber 8g

26 # grape celery power smoothie

Yield: 1 glass

Ingredients:
1. 1 cup black grapes.
2. 1 large stalk of celery
3. ½ cup instant oats
4. 1 tablespoon pumpkin seeds
5. ½ cup oat milk
6. ½ cup coconut water
7. ½ cup ice cubes

Preparation:
- Cut celery into 2-inch strips so it becomes easier to process.
- Put celery, oats, ice cubes and water in a blender and whiz on high speed until smooth. Add black grapes, pumpkin seed and milk blend until smooth.

- Pour into a glass and drink fresh.

Smoothie secret:
Believe it or not, coconut water has been administered to dehydrated patients via IV straight into their veins. This is because it is perfectly balanced to restore the body's fluids and is full of electrolytes. After a long day at work or a good workout, it's not uncommon to feel dehydrated. This soothing smoothie is the perfect way to replenish your body's water balance while indulging in a delicious treat. This smoothie also helps you with your joint pains, lung infections and asthma.

Nutritional information-

1. Calories = 266
2. Carbohydrate=19g
3. Protein =24g
4. Fiber 8g

27# Vanilla coconut green smoothie

Yield: 2 glasses

Ingredients:
1. 1 cup kale leaves
2. ½ cup Oats
3. ½ teaspoon vanilla extract
4. A pinch of salt
5. ¼ cup unsweetened coconut milk

6. ½ cup ice cubes

Preparation:
- Blend kale leaves and water first.
- When smooth, add oats, Vanilla extract, salt, coconut milk and ice cubes and blend until fully mixed.
- Pour into a glass and serve

Smoothie secret:

When you think of a powerhouse of nutrition, dark leafy greens always come to mind. They are a great source of vitamins like B, K, C, and E along with many essential minerals. This smoothie is a great one for those of you who are trying to become more accustomed to the flavor of greens. That's because I paired them up with tangy green and sweet vanilla for a smoothie that is green, but with a hint of sweetness.

Nutritional information-

1. Calories = 243
2. Carbohydrate=12g
3. Protein =11g
4. Fiber =8g

28# lemon forest green smoothie

Yield: 2 glasses

Ingredients:
- ½ cup pineapple
- ¼ cup cauliflower florets
- ½ cup pink grapefruit
- ½ tablespoon linseeds
- 1 tablespoon lemon zest
- ½ tablespoon almond nuts
- 2 tablespoon dried pitted dates (pre-soaked for a smoother blend)
- 1/4 cup dried apricots
- ½ cup non- dairy milk

Preparation:
1. Put water, milk, broccoli, Pineapple, cauliflower and grapefruit in a blender. Whiz until, mixed thoroughly.
2. Add linseeds, almonds, dates and apricots. Blend until smooth.
3. Pour into a tall glass and enjoy.

Smoothie secret:

Dreamy and creamy, this smoothie is like a melted Popsicle in a cup. And even though it's green, you'd never guess by its bright and fresh flavor that cauliflower florets have worked its way into the mix. Don't let the sweet, light flavor fool you either. This smoothie is packed with iron, protein, and fiber which make for a substantial drink.

Nutritional information-

1. Calories = 263
2. Carbohydrate=19g
3. Protein =34g
4. Fiber =8g

29# yogurt peach green smoothie

Yield: 2 glasses

Ingredients
1. 1 cup romaine lettuce
2. 3 small whole peaches
3. 1 tablespoon sesame seeds
4. ¼ cup dried apricots(pre-soaked for a smoother blend)
5. ½ cup non – dairy milk
6. ½ cup non-dairy yogurt
7. ½ cup ice cubes

Preparation:
- Blend in romaine lettuce, milk and yogurt until smooth.
- Add all remaining ingredients and process in the blender until thoroughly, mixed.
- Pour into a glass and drink immediately.

Smoothie secret:

For me, the heavy green flavor of dark leafy vegetables has been an acquired taste. That doesn't apply to this smoothie. Because of the addition of fresh flavors like dill, romaine lettuce, and citrus this smoothie is light and refreshing. It's a tasty combination that, if you are not a greens person, you will be glad you tried.

Nutritional information-

1. Calories = 276
2. Carbohydrate=53g
3. Protein =18g
4. Fiber =12g

30# green hurricane delta detox smoothie

Yield: 2 glasses

Ingredients
1. ½ cup spinach
2. ½ kale leaves
3. ¼ romaine lettuce
4. 4 broccoli heads
5. Medium stalk of celery
6. ¼ cup parsley leaves
7. ¼ cup Brussels sprouts
8. 5 mint leaves
9. 3 medium lemon
10. Pinch of sea salt
11. 1 cup ice cubes

Preparation:
- First peel lemon and square them.
- Put rest of the ingredient in the blender.
- Whiz until smooth
- Pour into glass and drink fresh.

Smoothie secret:

This smoothie is dedicated to all of the die-hard green smoothie addicts out there. This is the most hard core leafy green smoothie in this book. Please don't let that scare you off, though. The fresh lime lightens up the flavor quite a bit. There's even a bit of neutral zucchini thrown in the mix for a balanced, yet unmistakably green, drink.

Nutritional information-

1. Calories = 283
2. Carbohydrate=30g
3. Protein =30g
4. Fiber =47g

Conclusion

Getting healthy by eating plenty of smoothies filled with fruits, vegetables and protein is going to improve your health. You're going to love the way that these great smoothies taste and you're also going to absolutely love the way that each of them help you. Just take some time to make up these smoothies and you're going to be able to get started on healthy benefits. Your entire life is going to be a lot better if you just get started with this great, healthy diet. After all, you want to improve the way that all of your internal organs function and by implementing each of these different smoothies you're going to do just that for yourself

Going through a detox is going to be difficult for you but it's also going to be extremely important. A detox will allow you to correct your body and will definitely allow you to feel better throughout your life. With this detox program hopefully you'll be ready and able to accomplish even more in your own life. It's all about getting rid of the toxins that are slowing down your body and making sure that you get some great healthy foods in your system.

Take some time out of each day and make sure that you are watching out for your own health. Your detox, this detox plan, is going to allow you to get further in your life a lot faster. If you want to lose weight or you want to get in better shape just take the initiative. It's going to take a little effort but you're going to get to the great results that you want much faster than you may have thought possible. Don't be afraid to take this step, you're going to wonder why you didn't do it much sooner.

Now that you've got all this information it's time for you to get started. We wish you all the best of luck and we know that if you take care of yourself and you start implementing these smoothies you're going to succeed and get your body in the best shape it's ever been in. It's all about the vegetables and the great, healthy greens. With just a quality blender and a trip to the store for some healthy ingredients you'll be back on track before you even know it.